HEALTHY
HIGH-FIBER
COOKING

Cover Photo: Tropical Fruit Salad, page 48; Whole-Wheat French Bread, page 114;
Chicken-Vegetable Bake, page 70

HEALTHY
HIGH-FIBER
COOKING

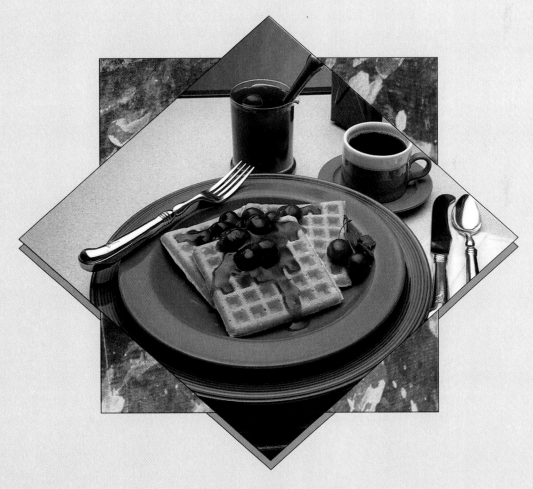

Jeanette P. Egan

Dedication

I would like to dedicate this book to my mother, Recie K. Parsons.

Acknowledgments

Special thanks to my husband, John H. Egan, for his vital role in seeing me through the writing of this book. I would also like to thank Lucy Thurston, Eleanor Carter, Patsy Brannon and Wesley Buchanan for their suggestions, help and moral support during this project.

ANOTHER BEST-SELLING VOLUME FROM HPBOOKS

Publisher: Rick Bailey
Executive Editor: Randy Summerlin
Editorial Director: Elaine R. Woodard
Editor: Patricia J. Aaron
Art Director: Don Burton
Book Design: Leslie Sinclair
Managing Editor: Cindy J. Coatsworth
Typography: Michelle Carter
Beverly Fine
Director of Manufacturing: Anthony B. Narducci
Photography & Food Styling: Burke/Triolo

Published by HPBooks, a division of HPBooks, Inc.
ISBN 0-89586-477-0
Library of Congress Catalog Card Number
©1987 HPBooks, Inc.   Printed in the U.S.A.
1st Printing

Notice: The information contained in this book is true and complete to the best of our knowledge. All recommendations are made without any guarantees on the part of the author or HPBooks. The author and publisher disclaim all liability in connection with the use of this information.

Some accessories for photography were from Mark Krasne, Inc. Los Angeles

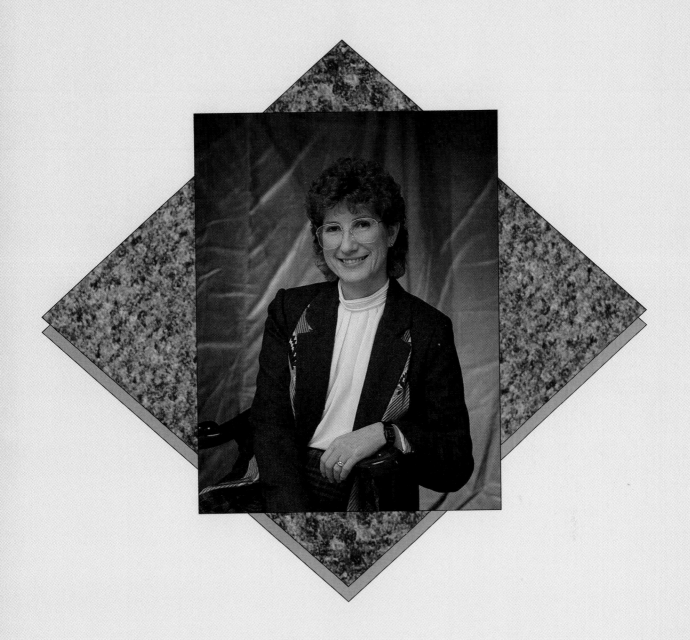

The benefits of a high fiber diet and the challenge of making wholesome foods taste and look delicious are of ongoing interest to Jeanette P. Egan. Having worked in public health nutrition as a counselor in weight control, diabetes, heart disease and other illnesses, she realized the need for delicious, appealing recipes with easy-to-obtain ingredients to motivate clients to improve their eating habits. Of particular interest to Jeanette is the relationship of diet to osteoporosis and cancer and the nutritional status of the elderly population. Holding degrees in Home Economics and Foods and Nutrition, she is a doctoral candidate in Nutrition and Food Science at the University of Arizona. Jeanette and husband John reside in Tucson, Arizona. Living in Germany for several years and traveling extensively contributed to the Egans' interest in new foods. They share hobbies of camping and traveling.

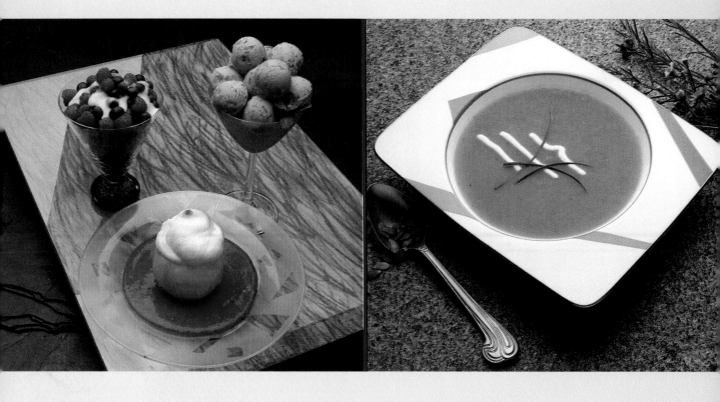

Contents

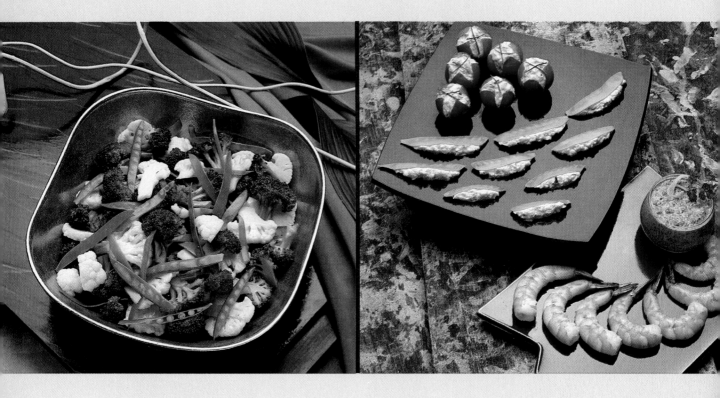

Introduction

Nutrition experts say that the American diet is too high in salt, sugar and fat. It is too low in fruits, vegetables and fiber. The Department of Agriculture and the National Cancer Institute tell us we may be able to reduce the rate of heart attack, stroke, high blood pressure and several types of cancer by just adjusting our eating habits. In addition we can reduce the effect of diabetes, osteoporosis and other illnesses that reduce the quality of life in our society.

The current interest in exercise and fitness emphasizes the need for changing our diets at the same time we change other aspects of our lifestyle. The question is how do we go about this without giving up the one thing most of us like best—TASTE. What is needed is not a diet book but a book designed to incorporate the latest ideas in healthy eating in tasty, easy-to-prepare recipes that will make you wonder why someone hasn't written a book like this before.

Fiber is "in"! Television commercials and magazine advertising attest to the interest in fiber. Within the last year, most of the major magazines have featured articles on fiber. Cereal companies have been quick to respond to the interest in fiber by introducing several high-fiber products that offer as much as 13 grams of fiber per serving.

Of course, our grandmothers knew that fiber—they called it roughage, was good for us. However, scientists were a little slow in catching up! During the last 10 years, researchers in the United States and Britain have been investigating the effects of high fiber diets on several diseases, such as diabetes, heart disease, high blood pressure, diverticulosis and even colon cancer. Recently several organizations, such as the National Cancer Institute, the American Heart Association, the Department of Health and Human Services and the Department of Agriculture have included an increased intake of fiber in their dietary recommendations.

What is dietary fiber?

Fiber is not one simple compound; it is made up of several different components. There are two basic types of dietary fiber—those that do not dissolve in water (insoluble) and those that do (soluble). The different methods for analyzing fiber in the laboratory give different results. Former methods discarded the soluble fiber and accounted only for part of the insoluble fiber. Early research in fiber concentrated on the insoluble form, because the methods of analysis did not detect soluble fiber. In 1984, an official method for fiber analysis was adopted by the Food and Drug Administration. It will take some time before all food composition tables reflect the changes. Many labels today still list crude fiber values instead of dietary fiber values. Because of the problems in analyzing fiber and because different fibers have different actions, it was originally difficult to determine the effects of fiber in the diet.

Dietary fiber only comes from plants. Just as plants contain no cholesterol, animal products contain no fiber. Fiber is the part of the plant that is not digested and absorbed in the small intestine. It passes into the large intestine (colon). What happens to fiber in the large intestine depends on its type.

Insoluble fibers absorb water and pass through the digestive system virtually unchanged. Soluble fibers may be broken down by bacteria in the large intestine into other substances. The exact mechanisms by which fiber works are not known. Because soluble and insoluble fiber have different actions in the body, it is important to eat foods containing both types.

Good sources of soluble fibers are beans, carrots, broccoli, apples, peaches, citrus fruits, oats and barley. Researchers are studying the role of soluble fiber in reducing cholesterol and blood sugar levels in diabetics with favorable results. Dr. James Anderson at the University of Kentucky and others have shown significant drops in blood cholesterol levels on diets high in soluble fibers. This may be important in treating patients with heart disease. So the adage "An apple a day, keeps the doctor away" may have a scientific basis.

Insoluble fiber is found in wheat bran, corn bran, dried beans and peas, nuts and most fruits and vegetables. Because insoluble fiber absorbs water, it increases bulk and thus acts as a natural laxative. Insoluble fiber is important in preventing diseases of the digestive system, such as diverticulosis (formation of small pouches on the walls of the intestine), constipation and hemorrhoids. There is epidemiological evidence that it may be important in preventing colon cancer.

Besides being important in disease prevention, high fiber foods are important in weight control. They promote a feeling of fullness and satisfaction, because the fiber absorbs water in the stomach and distends it. Foods high in soluble fiber tend to stay in the stomach longer, thus keeping you from being hungry. Both types of fiber slow down the absorption of glucose from the food; this prevents peaks in blood sugar and provides a steadier supply of energy. High fiber foods take longer to chew; this slows down the meal and allows the body time to be satiated without overeating. It's almost impossible to eat a crunchy salad or chewy brown rice in a hurry! In addition, fiber-rich foods usually contain fewer calories than foods that are low in fiber. Two exceptions to this are dried fruits and nuts. Go easy on these foods because they are relatively high in calories, especially the nuts. Ten to fifteen nuts can contain over 90 calories. The dried fruits are high in sugar and the nuts contain fat.

Why is fiber important in our diet?

Fiber is not considered an essential part of our diet the way vitamin C is. In case of a vitamin C deficiency, a recognized disease called scurvy develops that can only be cured by giving vitamin C. For fiber, there is no one disease that can be clearly said to result from the lack of fiber that can be cured by adding it to our diets (except for possibly constipation). However fiber seems to be necessary for the optimal functioning of our bodies. Research has shown that populations that have more fiber in the diet may have fewer of the debilitating diseases that populations with low fiber diets have. However, it is difficult to isolate one item as being the controlling factor, because these populations have many other things in their life and diet that are also different. Because a disease like cancer, for example, may take many years to develop, it is often difficult to

Fiber Content

Food	Insoluble Fiber (Grams)	Soluble Fiber (Grams)	
Asparagus, canned (1/2 cup)	🍎🍎	🍎	
Bean sprouts, raw (1 cup)	🍎🍎🍎	🍎	
Broccoli, cooked (1/2 cup)	🍎	🍎	
Brussel sprouts, cooked (1/2 cup)	🍎🍎▪	🍎🍎	
Carrots, cooked (1/2 cup)	🍎	🍎▪	
Cauliflower, cooked (1/2 cup)	🍎	▪	
Corn, cooked (1/2 cup)	🍎🍎	▪	
Eggplant, cooked (1/2 cup)	🍎▪	🍎	
Green beans, cooked (1/2 cup)	🍎🍎	🍎	
Peas, cooked (1/2 cup)	🍎🍎🍎	🍎	
Potatoes, mashed (1/2 cup)	🍎	🍎	
Pumpkin, canned (1/2 cup)	🍎🍎	🍎	
Spinach, cooked (1/2 cup)	🍎🍎	🍎	
Tomato, raw (1 medium)	🍎	▪	
Zucchini, cooked (1/2 cup)	🍎🍎	🍎▪	
Kidney beans, cooked (1/2 cup)	🍎🍎🍎🍎▪	🍎🍎🍎	
Lentils, cooked (1/2 cup)	🍎🍎🍎	🍎	
Pinto beans, cooked (1/2 cup)	🍎🍎🍎🍎	🍎🍎	
White beans, cooked (1/2 cup)	🍎🍎🍎🍎	🍎🍎	
Apple, raw (1 medium)	🍎🍎	🍎	
Apricots, raw (2)	🍎	🍎	
Banana, raw (1/2 medium)	🍎	▪	
Blueberries, raw (1/2 cup)	🍎🍎	▪	
Cantaloupe (1/4 small)	🍎	🍎	
Figs, dried (1 medium)	🍎🍎🍎	🍎	

1 🍎 = 1 gram fiber
1 🍎 = 3/4 gram fiber
1 🍎 = 1/2 gram fiber
1 🍎 = 1/4 gram fiber

Food	Insoluble Fiber (Grams)	Soluble Fiber (Grams)
Grapefruit, raw (1/2 medium)	🍎 (1/2)	🍎 (1)
Orange (1 small)	🍎 (1/2)	🍎 (3/4)
Pear, raw (1 medium)	🍎🍎🍎🍎 (3 3/4)	🍎 (3/4)
Pineapple, raw (1/2 cup)	🍎 (1)	🍎 (1/4)
Prunes, dried	🍎🍎🍎 (2 3/4)	🍎 (1)
Raisins (1 tablespoon)	🍎 (1/2)	🍎 (1/4)
Raspberries, raw (1/2 cup)	🍎🍎🍎🍎 (3 1/4)	🍎 (1/4)
Rhubarb, cooked (1/2 cup)	🍎 (1)	🍎 (1/2)
Strawberries, raw (1/2 cup)	🍎 (3/4)	🍎 (1/2)
Watermelon (1 cup)	🍎 (3/4)	🍎 (1/2)
Graham crackers (2 squares)	🍎 (1/2)	🍎 (1/2)
White bread (1 slice)	🍎 (1/4)	🍎 (1/4)
Whole-wheat bread (1 slice)	🍎🍎 (1 1/4)	🍎 (1/4)
Whole-wheat crackers (5)	🍎🍎 (1 1/2)	🍎 (1/2)
Brown rice (1/2 cup)	🍎 (3/4)	
Oat bran, uncooked (1/3 cup)	🍎🍎🍎 (2 1/4)	🍎🍎 (2)
Rolled oats, regular, cooked (3/4 cup)	🍎🍎 (1 1/2)	🍎🍎 (1 1/4)
Spaghetti, cooked (1/2 cup)	🍎 (1/2)	🍎 (1/4)
Wheat bran (1 tablespoon)	🍎🍎🍎🍎 (3 1/4)	🍎 (1/2)
Wheat germ (1 tablespoon)	🍎🍎 (1 1/4)	🍎 (1/4)
White rice (1/2 cup)	🍎 (1/4)	
Almonds, chopped (1 tablespoon)	🍎🍎 (2)	🍎 (1/4)
Pecans (2 whole)	🍎 (3/4)	🍎 (1/4)

Adapted from: Anderson, James W. *Plant Fiber in Foods*. 1986. HCF Diabetes Research Foundation, Inc. Used with permission.

pinpoint the exact cause. But there is enough evidence that fiber is important to our diets that nutritionists do recommend a diet that contains fiber from fruits, vegetables, beans and grains everyday.

What effect does cooking have on fiber?

Fiber does not seem to be destroyed by normal cooking methods. It may change form during toasting and browning. It may even seem to increase in toasted bread, but because bread also loses moisture during toasting it may be that there is only more fiber by dry weight! (This is similar to the false statement that toast has fewer calories than bread.) Fiber is affected by processing. During food preparation, the parts of the plant with the most fiber may be discarded, such as skins and bran.

How much fiber is enough?

The average American diet contains 10 to 20 grams of fiber per day. This is based on the data from the National Health and Nutrition Examination Survey II (NHANES II) and the National Cancer Institute (NCI). NCI recommends that we double our present intake; this would mean at least 20 to perhaps 40 grams per day. There is no Recommended Daily Allowance (RDA) for fiber as there is for calcium, for example. Increases in fiber should be from food rather than fiber supplements unless recommended by your doctor. It is not clear from the research available that you get the same beneficial effects from supplements that you do from food. Another reason for getting fiber from food is that in addition to fiber, you will be getting vitamins, minerals and other essential nutrients. No one who has any medical condition should change his or her diet without first consulting a doctor. This is especially true for diabetics,

because a high fiber diet may reduce insulin requirements.

How much is too much? Excess fiber may decrease the absorption of minerals and vitamins. But it is probably difficult, if not impossible, to get that much fiber from a high-fiber diet—another reason for not over-doing fiber supplements. For example, four bran muffins contain only 10 grams of fiber! Levels above 60 grams of fiber for an extended time might cause some nutritional deficiencies due to decreased absorption. If your doctor has you on a very high fiber diet, ask if you need to take vitamin or mineral supplements.

How should fiber be increased?

It is very important to slowly increase fiber-rich foods. This prevents any discomfort due to gas or bloating because of the formation of intestinal gas by the bacteria found in the large intestine. Increase fiber intake over a period of three or four weeks by making a few changes at a time. Eat whole-wheat bread and brown rice instead of white bread and white rice. Switch to whole-grain cereals. Check labels to see if your breads and cereals list the amount of dietary fiber. Some brown bread is just that—it's brown because of coloring agents, not whole-grain flour. Eat whole fruits, including the skin, instead of just drinking the juice. Eat more vegetables, fruits and whole-grain cereals. Include dried beans and legumes in your diet; they're good sources of both soluble and insoluble fiber.

Other Dietary Recommendations

Because fiber is only one constituent of food, it is necessary to balance our diets. Several government agencies have guidelines for healthy eating. In the table below are the Dietary Guidelines for Americans that were updated in 1985 by the U.S. Department of Agriculture and the U.S. Department of Health and Human Services.

Dietary Guidelines for Americans

1. **Eat a variety of foods**
2. **Maintain desirable weight**
3. **Avoid too much fat, saturated fat and cholesterol**
4. **Eat foods with adequate starch and fiber**
5. **Avoid too much sugar**
6. **Avoid too much sodium**
7. **If you drink alcoholic beverages, do so in moderation**

Home and Garden Bulletin No. 232

What do these guidelines mean? Let's take them in order. It's important to eat a variety of foods each day to insure adequate amounts of each of the approximately 40 nutrients. No one food alone supplies all of these, and besides, there may be some nutrients that we haven't discovered yet. The easiest way to eat a variety of foods is to choose foods from each of the food groups. They are: fruits and vegetables; breads and cereals; milk and dairy products; and meat and meat substitutes, such as dried beans and nuts.

What is meant by desirable weight? It's the weight that is right for you. Height and weight tables are one way of determining ideal body weight, but it may not be the most accurate. Consult a doctor or registered dietitian for additional information, if needed. Obesity may lead to serious medical problems, such as high blood pressure and diabetes. Even though being overweight may be dangerous, losing weight too rapidly may be even more so. If you need to lose weight, choose a well-balanced diet that lets you lose one to two pounds per week.

Fat supplies approximately 40 percent of the calories in the American diet. The National Cancer Institute and the American Heart Association both suggest that calories from fat be reduced to 30 percent. Fats contain over twice as many calories as protein and carbohydrates. (Nine calories per gram as compared to four calories for proteins and carbohydrates.) Excess dietary fat has been linked with certain types of cancer. High levels of saturated fat may increase blood cholesterol levels. Earlier there was more of an emphasis on polyunsaturated fats. Now experts suggest that equal amounts of saturated, monosaturated and polyunsaturated fats be consumed. Saturated fats are solid at room temperature; monosaturated fats and polyunsaturated fats are liquid at room temperature. Animal fats, coconut oil, palm oil and cocoa butter are saturated. Olive oil is a monosaturated fat. Corn oil and safflower oil are examples of polyunsaturated oils. Fish oils are receiving a lot of attention because of their high levels of omega-3 fatty acids. These fatty acids may be important in preventing several of the degenerative conditions, such as heart disease. It's best to get fish oils by eating fish at least three times per week.

It is suggested that 45 to 50 percent of the calories in our diets come from complex carbohydrates. Complex carbohydrates are starches that must be broken down into simple sugars before being absorbed into the body. Choose whole grains, fruits, vegetables, dry beans and peas. These foods contain vitamins, minerals and fiber as well as carbohydrates for energy.

Only about 10 percent of our calories should be from simple sugars, such as white sugar, brown sugar, honey and fructose. Simple sugars promote dental caries. The more often sugar is eaten, the greater the chance of tooth decay. Much of the sugar in our diets is hidden; check labels for corn syrup and word ending in "ose", such as dextrose, glucose and maltose.

Sodium is another hidden ingredient in much of our processed food. Together sodium and chlorine combine to make sodium chloride, common table salt—one of the most frequently used food additives! Too much salt or sodium may cause high blood pressure in susceptible individuals. Avoid salt substitutes unless suggested by your doctor. They don't taste the same as real salt so you'll have to become accustomed to the strange flavor. To reduce sodium intake, season foods with herbs, vinegar, lemon juice or wine. Always taste food before adding salt. Check labels for sodium, not just salt. If you do have a problem with high blood pressure, it's important to follow your doctor's orders.

The last guideline concerns alcohol consumption. Moderate consumption means two or less standard-size drinks per day. Because alcoholic drinks are high in calories, they can contribute a significant number of calories with few nutrients. Alcohol contains seven calories per gram—almost as much as fat. Dieters beware! Excess alcohol consumption may lead to nutritional deficiencies and serious illnesses.

Recommendations from the National Cancer Institute are similar to many of the Dietary Guidelines for Americans. They include: Eat foods low in fat, eat foods high in fiber, eat fresh fruits and vegetables, eat a balanced diet and be neither under or over weight.

As indicated by the suggestions from the different organizations, optimal health does not depend on merely increasing or decreasing one aspect of your diet. It is important to eat a well-balanced diet—something that you were taught along with the Basic Four in elementary school! However, from within those basic groups it is important to choose wisely. Selecting calories is like investing money, pick those foods whose calories pay the maximum return. While every investment doesn't have to pay a large dividend, the bottom line must be positive or the investor will soon have a deficient.

I would like to call attention to one of the most ignored nutrients—water! Water is important in any diet—remember the six to eight glasses a day, but it is especially important in a high-fiber diet. Fiber needs ample amounts of water to work effectively.

In addition to having a healthy diet, it's important to exercise regularly. Exercise helps reduce stress and burns up calories. One common ailment in older women, osteoporosis, is related to lack of exercise as well as several other factors, including not enough calcium in the diet.

About the Recipes

Recipes in this book were developed to contain both soluble and insoluble forms of fiber. A conscious effort was made to reduce salt, sugar and fat in the recipes without sacrificing taste. I enjoyed the amazed comments of our friends (all of whom cheerfully agreed to be "guinea pigs") when they tasted the dishes. "Do you mean this is GOOD for me? It's delicious!" One person even asked for a recipe so she could make it to impress her mother-in-law! So forget the idea that all fiber-rich foods taste like straw and contain wheat bran. While wheat bran is an important source of fiber, it is not the only one.

All recipes were analyzed for calorie and

fiber content. If an ingredient is listed as "if desired," then it is not included in the analysis. If a recipe make 4 to 6 servings, the analysis is based on 4 servings. If you serve the dish to six people, each will get slightly fewer calories and fiber than that listed for the recipe. Because the analysis of fiber in food is just now being standardized, there will be some variation between different sources. Early fiber analysis gave values for crude fiber, underestimating soluble fiber. Values in this book are based on dietary fiber. If you find a label that still lists crude fiber, you can multiply it by four to get an estimated dietary fiber value.

The amount of salt in all recipes except baked goods is left to the discretion of the cook. I would suggest that you add about half what you think is needed and then taste before adding more. Dishes can be tasted for seasonings before serving and adjusted if necessary. Taste for hot-pepper sauce, herbs and vinegar, too. The amounts listed are to my taste; you may prefer more or less.

To further reduce cholesterol in these recipes, egg substitutes could be used instead of eggs. However, if you must reduce sodium intake, check the labels for sodium content before making the substitution. All recipes call for either butter or margarine; use your own judgement when deciding which to add. Unsalted butter or margarine can be used to reduce the sodium content of recipes. It's important to store unsalted butter or margarine in the freezer; leave only the amount in the refrigerator that will be eaten within a few days to prevent development of off flavors.

Use nonstick pans to reduce amounts of fat needed to prevent sticking. Nonstick cooking spray is another way to reduce calories from fat; I prefer to use spray in a pump bottle rather than the aerosol can.

Cooking Hints

Steam vegetables only until crisp-tender to conserve vitamins; season with herbs or lemon juice instead of butter or margarine. Never add baking soda to green vegetables to preserve the bright green color; it destroys vitamins. Instead, always bring the water to a boil first, then add the vegetables to the steamer. Cook without a lid for a few minutes, then cover for the remaining cooking time. This method and not overcooking will ensure bright green vegetables every time. Stir-frying in a small amount of fat or boiling in a small amount of water are other ways to retain the water-soluble vitamins in vegetables. Prepare vegetables just before cooking. Leaving cut-up foods on the countertop will destroy their vitamin C content, as will overcooking.

To ensure success when cooking, always read the recipe through completely before starting to cook, then check that you have all the necessary ingredients. Each recipe usually lists a cooking time and then tells what should happen. For example, bake about 30 minutes or until top of cake springs back when lightly pressed. Because ovens vary, check before the 30 minutes are up to see if what is supposed to happen has, in this case, if the top of the cake springs back. If not, bake about 5 minutes more or until done.

Sodium & Salt

If you need to reduce the amount of salt that you eat, there are several products to help you. In addition to the low-sodium broths and soy sauce, there are other products with reduced sodium available. These include nuts, salad dressings, mayonnaise, ketchup, tomato sauce, canned vegetables, vegetable juices, cereals, corn chips, potato chips and soups. (It's a list that literally includes everything from soups to nuts!) Plain frozen vegetables are good choices, because, except for peas and lima beans, which use salt during processing, they have no added salt. As these products are usually stocked along with the regular versions in your supermarket, it's important to read labels.

Because it is sometimes difficult to understand the wording on labels the following box should help.

Labeling for Salt & Sodium

Based on guidelines passed by the Food and Drug Administration (FDA) in 1984, the following terms apply to salt and sodium when labeling products.

No sodium or sodium free: Less than 5 mg sodium per serving.

Very low sodium: 35 mg sodium or less per serving.

Low sodium: 140 mg sodium or less per serving.

Reduced sodium: Sodium content reduced by 75 percent as compared with a standard similar product prepared with salt.

Unsalted: Food product processed without salt, but one that would usually be salted, such as unsalted tomato sauce.

Anyone who has a chronic health problem, such as diabetes, or is on a special diet should consult his or her physician before making major dietary changes. This is not a diet book but a collection of recipes designed to include higher amounts of fiber and lower amounts of fat, sugar and salt.

Breakfast

	Calories	Fiber (grams)	Cholesterol (milligrams)
1 medium-size banana	32	0.5	0
1 cup strawberries	56	3.3	0
1/2 cup My Muesli, page 132	205	3.6	0
1 cup low-fat milk	122	0.0	20
TOTAL	**415**	**7.4**	**20**
1/2 medium-size grapefruit	40	1.7	0
1 serving Spinach Frittata with Herbed Tomato Sauce, page 134	155	2.6	138
2 toasted Oat Bread slices, page 117	234	5.2	17
1 cup low-fat milk	122	0.0	20
TOTAL	**551**	**9.5**	**195**
1/4 medium-size cantaloupe	30	1.6	0
1 Whole-Wheat Waffle, page 129	179	2.0	72
1/3 cup Blueberry-Orange Sauce, page 130	30	0.6	0
TOTAL	**418**	**6.2**	**72**

Lunch

	Calories	Fiber (grams)	Cholesterol (milligrams)
1 serving Chicken-Melon Salad, page 57	384	1.7	78
2 Banana-Marmalade Muffins, page 124	320	4.4	46
1 cup low-fat milk	122	0.0	20
1 medium-size orange	70	1.5	0
TOTAL	**896**	**7.6**	**144**
1 serving Lentil-Vegetable Soup, page 41	195	3.1	1
4 whole-wheat crackers	64	1.3	0
1 cup low-fat milk	122	0.0	20
1 medium-size apple	87	2.8	0
TOTAL	**468**	**7.2**	**21**
1 serving Quick Double-Corn Chowder, page 42	155	2.4	26
2 Wheat-Berry Bread slices, page 113	220	4.6	0.3
1/2 medium-size green bell pepper	11	1.0	0
2 medium-size celery stalks	16	1.2	0
1 cup low-fat milk	122	0.0	20
1 Applesauce-Fig Bar, page 156	101	1.3	22
TOTAL	**625**	**10.5**	**68.3**

Dinner

	Calories	Fiber (grams)	Cholesterol (milligrams)
1 serving Eggplant Casserole, page 64	247	4.8	48
1 serving Garden Salad, page 56	106	1.9	0
1 round Middle Eastern Flat Bread, page 115	150	4.0	0
1 serving Mango Sorbet, page 151	75	1.4	0
TOTAL	**578**	**12.1**	**48**
1 serving Oven-Fried Chicken, page 72	210	3.6	80
1 serving Green Beans & Potatoes, page 85	205	3.7	0
1 serving Broiled Tomato with Dill-Mustard Sauce, page 92	243	1.7	12
1 serving "Green" Salad, page 52	129	2.6	0
1 serving Melon Cup, page 48	36	0.5	0
TOTAL	**823**	**12.1**	**92**
1 serving Spinach-Stuffed Fish Fillets, page 80	201	0.9	70
1/2 cup Basic Brown Rice, page 103	112	0.7	0
1 serving Carrot Salad, page 54	141	1.8	0
1 serving Creamy Berry Dessert, page 144	273	5.1	142
TOTAL	**756**	**9.3**	**212**

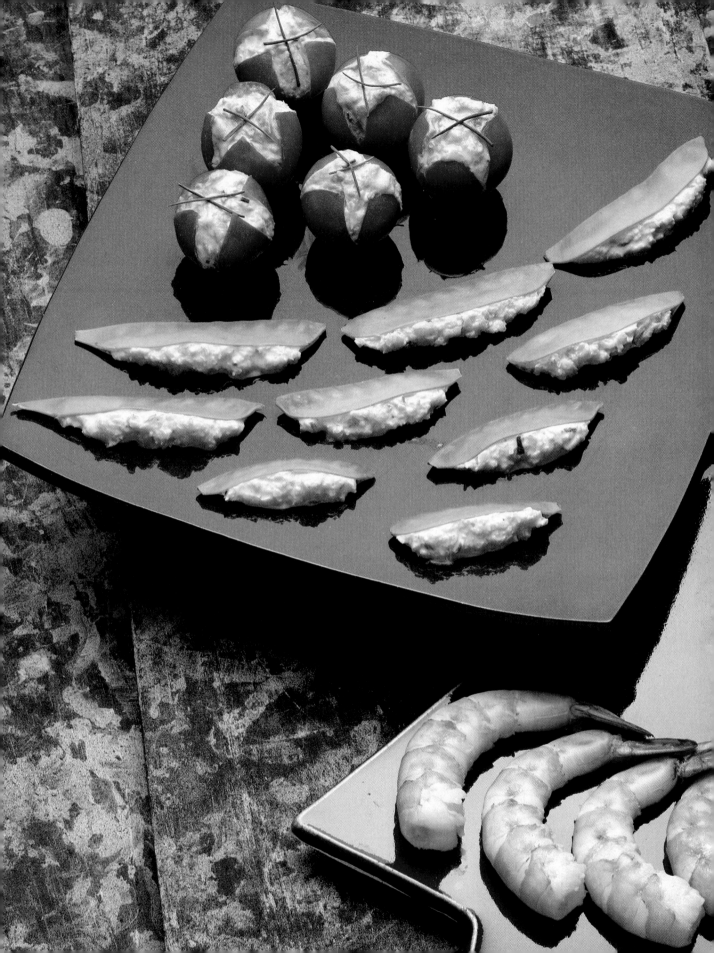

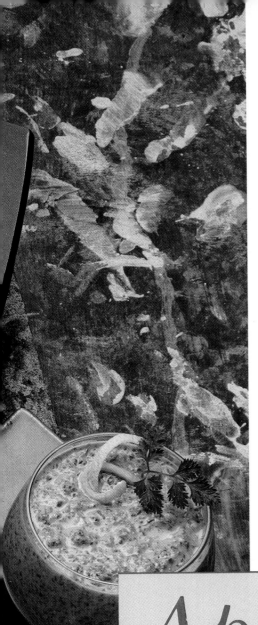

Clockwise from top left: Salmon-Filled Cherry Tomatoes, page 23;
Shrimp Stuffed Peapods, page 23; Pesto Spinach Dip with shrimp,
page 30

Appetizers & Snacks

CHAPTER ONE

Appetizers
& Snacks

Appetizers and snacks add interest to our daily diet. They fill gaps between meals or may even substitute for a meal. However, appetizers and snacks are often not considered when planning food intake for the day. Yet they can contribute important nutrients missed at meals. Planned unwisely, appetizers and snacks can be a major source of empty calories—calories without much in the way of vitamins and minerals. Some sweets and soft drinks fall into this category. So is snacking a bad habit? Maybe—you see it depends on the snack!

A healthy snack may be as simple as a crisp apple or a refreshing glass of orange juice. Or by planning ahead, you can have Blueberry-Banana Pops, page 33, or Cheesy Popcorn, page 33. Popped corn only takes minutes and is a good source of fiber. Just go easy on the butter and salt.

When planning appetizers for a party, remember the same guidelines that you would in planning a menu for a meal—think variety. Provide diversity in flavors, textures, temperatures, colors and shapes. Provide dishes for those friends who are on special diets or just watching calories. Raw vegetables are excellent high-fiber, low-calorie choices. Serve them alone or with one of the hot or cold dips in this chapter.

Beverages, such as the ones in this chapter, are often used as snacks by themselves. However, beverages are often served with appetizers and snacks. Some choices in beverages include juices, mineral water, tea and coffee. There is a trend towards lighter alcoholic and nonalcoholic drinks. If you're serving alcoholic drinks, choose a light wine or punch. Always offer nonalcoholic drinks, such as juices or mineral water, for those people who do not want to drink alcoholic beverages. Remember that alcohol contributes seven calories per gram; this is more than any food except fats and oils. Conversely, researchers have found that those who drink only one or two alcoholic drinks a day may live longer and be healthier in general than those who don't drink or those who drink more than two drinks a day.

So remember, plan healthy appetizers and snacks as part of your overall eating plan. Healthy doesn't mean boring!

Salmon-Filled Cherry Tomatoes

Add a touch of color to your table with these tempting appetizers. (Photo on page 20.)

1 pint cherry tomatoes (about 22)
1 (6-oz.) can salmon, drained, flaked
1 (3-oz.) package Neufchâtel cheese,
  room temperature
1 tablespoon lemon juice
1 tablespoon chopped chives

1/2 teaspoon dried leaf tarragon,
  if desired
Salt
Freshly ground pepper
Chopped fresh parsley if desired
Chives, if desired

Cut a thin slice off stem end of each tomato. Using a small spoon or grapefruit knife, remove and discard tomato pulp. Drain tomatoes upside down on paper towels. In a medium-size bowl, combine salmon, cheese, lemon juice, chives and tarragon, if desired, until salmon is finely flaked. Season with salt and pepper. Stuff tomatoes with salmon mixture. Cover and refrigerate until chilled or up to 8 hours. To serve, garnish with parsley and chives, if desired. Makes about 22 appetizers.

Per appetizer:
20 calories
0.2 gram fiber

Shrimp & Cucumber Bites

The crunchy cucumber and creamy filling complement each other. (Photo on page 20.)

6 ounces peeled cooked shrimp
1 green onion, coarsely chopped
1 large celery stalk, chopped
3 tablespoons plain low-fat yogurt
2 tablespoons mayonnaise
1 tablespoon lemon juice

2 teaspoons green-peppercorn mustard
Salt
Freshly ground pepper
2 large cucumbers
Paprika

In a food processor fitted with the metal blade, combine shrimp, green onion, celery, yogurt, mayonnaise, lemon juice and mustard. Process just until shrimp are coarsely chopped; do not overprocess. Season with salt and pepper; set aside. Using tines of a fork, score cucumbers lengthwise. Cut off and discard ends. Cut cucumbers crosswise in 3/4-inch slices. Using a small melon baller or small spoon, scoop out centers of cucumbers leaving 1/4-inch bottoms. Fill centers with shrimp mixture. Cover and refrigerate until ready to serve or up to 6 hours. Sprinkle with paprika. Makes about 30 appetizers.

Per appetizer:
32 calories
0.5 gram fiber

Variation
Shrimp Stuffed Peapods: Substitute about 30 Chinese peapods for cucumber. Slit peapods open along straight edge. Fill with shrimp mixture.

Roasted Peppers

You'll find many ways to use this dish. Serve alone, as part of an antipasto selection or as a sandwich topping.

1 large red bell pepper
1 large green bell pepper
1 teaspoon dried leaf basil
1/2 teaspoon dried leaf oregano

Salt
Freshly ground pepper
2 tablespoons white-wine vinegar
1 tablespoon olive oil

Per serving:
41 calories
0.5 gram fiber

Position oven rack 4 to 6 inches from heat source. Preheat broiler. Broil peppers in preheated oven, turning frequently, 15 minutes or until skins are blistered. Steam in a paper bag or foil 15 minutes. When cool enough to handle, peel and core peppers. Discard skin and seeds. Cut lengthwise in 1/4-inch strips. Arrange strips in a shallow bowl. Sprinkle with basil and oregano. Season with salt and pepper. In a small bowl, whisk vinegar and olive oil until slightly thickened; drizzle over pepper strips. Cover and let stand 1 hour before serving, or refrigerate up to 2 days. Serve at room temperature. Makes 4 servings.

Roasted Pepper & Ham Appetizers

This is delicious with roast turkey. It can also be served as four open-faced sandwiches.

Dijon-style mustard
4 slices whole-wheat bread
4 (1-oz.) lean ham slices

1 recipe Roasted Peppers, above
1 cup (4 oz.) shredded part-skim
    mozzarella cheese

Per appetizer:
62 calories
0.3 gram fiber

Position oven rack 4 to 6 inches from heat source. Preheat broiler. Spread mustard on 1 side of bread. Place, mustard-side up, on a baking sheet. Top with ham slices. Spoon peppers on ham slices. Sprinkle with cheese. Broil in preheated oven until cheese melts. Cut each sandwich in 4 quarters. Makes 16 appetizers.

Mediterranean Vegetable Appetizer

Serve warm or at room temperature with crisp whole-wheat lavosh or raw vegetables.

1 large eggplant, cubed
1 large garlic clove, minced
1 small onion, finely chopped
4 ounces mushrooms, chopped
1 small zucchini, chopped
1 large tomato, chopped
1/2 cup dry white wine

1 teaspoon dried leaf basil
1 teaspoon dried leaf oregano
Salt
Freshly ground pepper
2 tablespoons grated Parmesan cheese,
    if desired

I n a medium-size saucepan, combine eggplant, garlic, onion, mushrooms, zucchini, tomato, wine, basil and oregano. Season with salt and pepper. Bring to a boil. Reduce heat, cover and simmer, gently stirring occasionally, 20 minutes or until vegetables are tender and beginning to lose their shapes. Cool; sprinkle with cheese, if desired. Makes 3 cups.

Per 1/4 cup:
45 calories
2.2 grams fiber

Potato Skins

A delicious and nutritious high-fiber snack. These are baked, not fried.

4 medium-size baking potatoes,
    scrubbed, pierced
1/4 cup shredded lean ham
1/4 cup shredded cooked chicken
1 cup (4 oz.) shredded part-skim
    mozzarella cheese

1 tablespoon capers, drained, chopped
1 tablespoon chopped fresh parsley
1 tablespoon low-fat milk
Salt
Freshly ground pepper

P reheat oven to 375F (190C). Bake potatoes in preheated oven 1 hour or until fork-tender. Cool until potatoes can be handled. Cut in half lengthwise. Scoop out pulp leaving a 1/4- to 1/2-inch shell. Reserve pulp for another use. Position oven rack 4 to 6 inches from heat source. Preheat broiler. In a medium-size bowl, combine ham, chicken, cheese, capers, parsley and milk. Season with salt and pepper. Spoon mixture into potato shells. Broil until hot and bubbly. Makes 8 appetizers.

Per appetizer:
100 calories
1.4 grams fiber

Sausage Potatoes

Cook these easy appetizers ahead and reheat before serving.

30 (about 1-1/2-inch in diameter) new
   red potatoes

10 ounces turkey sausage
1 cup (4 oz.) shredded Cheddar cheese

Preheat oven to 425F (220C). Grease bottom of a 13" x 9" baking pan. Cut a thin slice off top of each potato. Using a small melon baller, remove and discard 1 scoop of each potato. Stuff each potato cavity with sausage. Place in greased baking pan. Bake in preheated oven 30 minutes or until potatoes are tender when pierced with a fork. Sprinkle with cheese. Bake 5 minutes or until cheese melts. Serve hot. Makes 30 appetizers.

Feta Cheese Appetizers

I first ate these appetizers at a Greek restaurant in Germany. Experimentation provided this recipe!

4 ounces feta cheese, drained, rinsed,
   cut in 1/4-inch slices
1 teaspoon olive oil
1 large onion, thinly sliced
2 teaspoons dried leaf oregano

1 teaspoon ground cumin
Freshly ground pepper
2 whole-wheat pita bread rounds or
   Middle Eastern Flat Bread, page 115,
   cut in 8 wedges

Preheat oven to 425F (220C). Cut a foil sheet about 15 inches in length. Place cheese in center of foil; set aside. In a medium-size skillet, heat olive oil over medium heat. Add onion. Cook, stirring occasionally, until softened. Spoon onions over cheese. Sprinkle with oregano and cumin. Season with pepper. Tightly seal edges of foil. Place package on a baking sheet. Bake in preheated oven 20 minutes or until cheese is softened. (Carefully open foil to check.) Spoon cheese and juices into a heated serving dish. Serve with bread. Makes 4 servings.

Quesadillas

Quick and easy to make, this can also be served as a light meal.

2 (10-inch) flour tortillas
1 cup (4 oz.) shredded part-skim
   mozzarella cheese
1 large onion, thinly sliced
1 (4-oz.) can green chilies, drained, cut
   lengthwise in julienne strips

1/4 cup chopped fresh cilantro or
   fresh basil
Freshly ground pepper

Preheat a griddle over medium heat. Sprinkle 1 tortilla with cheese, onion, chilies and cilantro. Season with pepper. Place on preheated griddle. Top with remaining tortilla. Cook until cheese melts, turning over once. Cut in 8 wedges. Makes 8 appetizers.

**Per appetizer:
100 calories
1.5 grams fiber**

Quick Pizza

Pizza can be suprisingly high in fiber. For a thinner crust, split the flat bread in half.

1 tablespoon olive oil
1/2 medium-size green bell pepper,
   thinly sliced
1 small onion, thinly sliced
1/2 cup crushed Italian-style tomatoes
1 teaspoon dried leaf basil
1 teaspoon dried leaf oregano
1/4 teaspoon crushed caraway seeds

Hot-pepper sauce
Salt
Freshly ground pepper
2 rounds Middle Eastern Flat Bread,
   page 115, or 2 pita bread rounds
1 cup (4 oz.) shredded part-skim
   mozzarella cheese

Preheat oven to 425F (220C). In a small skillet, heat olive oil over medium heat. Add bell pepper and onion; cook until softened. In a small bowl, combine tomatoes, basil, oregano and caraway seeds. Season with hot-pepper sauce, salt and pepper. Place bread on a baking sheet. Spoon tomato mixture over bread rounds. Top with bell pepper and onion. Sprinkle with cheese. Bake in preheated oven 5 minutes or until cheese melts and topping is bubbly. Makes 2 servings.

**Per serving:
170 calories
1.7 grams fiber**

Patsy's Gingery Pot Stickers

Turkey sausage is a suprise ingredient.

1 small zucchini, finely shredded
8 ounces turkey sausage
1 tablespoon minced ginger root
3/4 teaspoon reduced-sodium soy sauce
3/4 teaspoon dry sherry
1-1/2 tablespoons cornstarch

Cooking Sauce:
4 thin slices ginger root
2/3 cup sherry

Dipping Sauce:
2 tablespoons reduced-sodium soy sauce
1/4 cup seasoned rice vinegar

2 tablespoons unprocessed wheat bran
1 (12-oz.) package pot-sticker or won-ton
    wrappers, separated
Water
Cornstarch
2 tablespoons vegetable oil

2/3 cup water

1/2 teaspoon finely minced garlic

Prepare Cooking Sauce; set aside. Prepare Dipping Sauce; set aside. In a medium-size bowl, combine zucchini, sausage, ginger root, soy sauce, sherry, cornstarch and wheat bran. Place 1 teaspoon of filling in center of each wrapper. Lightly moisten 1/2 of outer wrapper edge with water. Fold in half, sealing edges. Make 5 to 6 pleats along sealed edge. Lightly dust a large plate with cornstarch. Place pot stickers on plate with pleated-edges upright. In a 9-inch skillet, heat 1 tablespoon of oil over medium-high heat. When hot, reduce heat to medium. Arrange 25 pot stickers, pleated-edges up, in skillet. Cook 3 to 4 minutes or until bottoms are lightly browned. Add 1/2 of Cooking Sauce. Cover and cook 10 to 12 minutes or until sauce evaporates. Place pot stickers on a serving plate; keep warm. Repeat with remaining pot stickers and cooking sauce. Discard ginger root. Serve with Dipping Sauce. Makes about 50 pot stickers.

Cooking Sauce:
In a 2-cup glass measure, combine ginger root, sherry and water.

Dipping Sauce:
In a small serving bowl, combine soy sauce, vinegar and garlic.

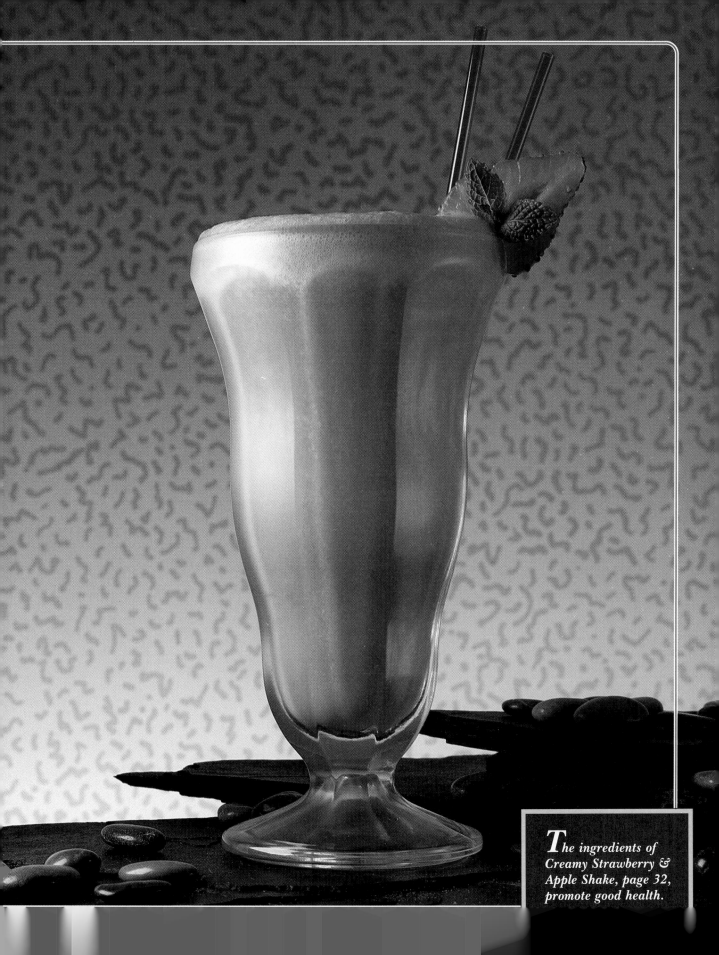

*T*he ingredients of *Creamy Strawberry & Apple Shake, page 32,* promote good health.

Easy Garbanzo-Bean Dip

The sesame flavor is from sesame oil rather than the traditional tahini or sesame-seed paste. Serve with pita-bread wedges or raw vegetables.

1 (15-oz.) can garbanzo beans, drained	Salt
2 to 3 tablespoons lemon juice	White pepper
1 large garlic clove, chopped	1 medium-size tomato, chopped
1 teaspoon sesame oil	1 tablespoon minced fresh parsley
Hot-pepper sauce	Paprika

In a food processor fitted with the metal blade, combine beans, lemon juice, garlic and sesame oil. Process to a puree. Season with hot-pepper sauce, salt and white pepper. Add tomato and parsley; process just until tomato is finely chopped. Spoon into a serving bowl. Sprinkle with paprika. Makes about 2 cups.

Pesto Spinach Dip

Serve with cooked shrimp or raw vegetables. (Photo on page 20.)

1 bunch spinach, trimmed, coarsely chopped	2 tablespoons grated Parmesan cheese
1/2 cup plain low-fat yogurt	1 tablespoon olive oil
1/4 cup walnuts	Salt
2 tablespoons chopped fresh basil or 2 teaspoons dried leaf basil	Freshly ground pepper
	Strip lemon peel, if desired
	Cilantro sprig, if desired

In a food processor fitted with the metal blade, place spinach, yogurt, walnuts, basil, cheese and olive oil. Season with salt and pepper. Process until combined. Pour into a small serving dish. Cover and refrigerate at least 2 hours or up to 8 hours. To serve, garnish with lemon peel and cilantro, if desired. Makes about 1 cup.

Variation
Substitute tarragon or cilantro for basil.

Hot & Spicy Bean Dip

Serve this quick and easy dip with tortilla chips or raw vegetables.

1 (15-oz.) can vegetarian-style refried
   beans or "Refried" Beans, page 99
1 cup prepared picante sauce
1 teaspoon chili powder

1/2 teaspoon ground cumin
Hot-pepper sauce
1/2 cup (2 oz.) shredded Monterey Jack
   cheese

In a medium-size saucepan, combine beans, picante sauce, chili powder and cumin. Season with hot-pepper sauce. Cook, stirring constantly, over medium heat until hot and bubbly. Spoon into a serving dish. Sprinkle with cheese. Makes 8 servings.

Per serving:
80 calories
2.0 grams fiber

Southwest Bean Appetizer

High in fiber and flavor, this traditional southwestern dish is great served with corn chips, jicama or carrot slices.

1 (15-oz.) can vegetarian-style refried
   beans or 2 cups "Refried" Beans,
   page 99
1/2 medium-size onion, finely chopped
1 (4-oz.) can diced green chilies, drained
1 teaspoon ground cumin

1 cup (4 oz.) shredded Monterey Jack
   cheese
1 cup Salsa, below, or prepared picante
   sauce or salsa
1 large tomato, chopped
2 cups shredded iceberg lettuce

Preheat oven to 350F (175C). Grease a shallow 12-inch-round baking dish. In a medium-size bowl, combine beans, onion, chilies and cumin. Spread mixture in greased dish. Sprinkle with cheese. Bake in preheated oven 20 minutes or until mixture is hot and cheese is melted. Pour salsa over cheese. Arrange tomatoes and lettuce around appetizer. Makes 8 servings.

Per serving:
108 calories
1.5 grams fiber

Salsa

Use this New Mexican-style salsa to top everything from omelets to baked chicken, or serve as a dip with crisp tortillas.

1 pound tomatoes, chopped
1 medium-size red onion, finely
   chopped
1 (4-oz.) can diced green chilies, drained

1/4 cup packed finely chopped fresh
   cilantro
1 tablespoon white-wine vinegar
Salt

In a medium-size bowl, combine tomatoes, onion, chilies, cilantro and vinegar. Season with salt. Cover and refrigerate until chilled. Makes about 4 cups.

Per 1/4 cup:
15 calories
0.5 gram fiber

Peach-Apricot Shake

This shake has a rich fruity flavor. For a smoother texture, soak the apricots in the apple juice about 10 minutes before processing.

1/2 cup chopped dried apricots
1/2 cup unsweetened apple juice

1 cup peach sorbet
1 cup low-fat milk

In a blender, process apricots and apple juice to a puree. Add sorbet and milk. Process until combined. Makes 2 servings.

Creamy Strawberry & Apple Shake

My husband created this refreshing drink! (Photo on page 29.)

2 cups fresh or thawed frozen
   strawberries
1 cup plain low-fat yogurt
2-1/2 cups unsweetened apple juice,
   chilled

1 fresh strawberry, cut in half, if desired
Mint sprig, if desired

In a blender, process strawberries, yogurt and apple juice 1 minute or until smooth. Garnish with strawbery and mint, if desired. Makes 2 servings.

Variation
Add 1 chopped ripe banana to above ingredients. If mixture is too thick, add more apple juice. Makes 2 to 3 servings.

Blackberry-Apple Shake

A great summertime drink when blackberries are ripe.

2 cups fresh or frozen blackberries
1 cup unsweetened apple juice
1 cup plain low-fat yogurt

1 tablespoon honey
1/2 cup crushed ice, if desired

In a blender, process blackberries, apple juice, yogurt, honey and ice, if desired, until combined. Makes 4 servings.

Blueberry-Banana Pops

Refreshing and easy to do! Plastic holders for freezing pops are available.

3 medium-size very ripe bananas,
  mashed
1 cup fresh or thawed frozen blueberries

1 tablespoon honey
1 teaspoon vanilla extract

In a blender or a food processor fitted with the metal blade, process bananas, blueberries, honey and vanilla to a puree. Pour into 9 (3-oz.) paper cups or plastic holders, filling each cup about 2/3 full. Freeze 1 hour or until partially frozen. Insert a plastic spoon or a wooden ice-cream stick in center of each pop. Freeze 2 hours more or until firm. To serve, peel off paper cups or remove from plastic holders. Makes 9 pops.

**Per pop:
51 calories
1.0 gram fiber**

Peachy Yogurt Pops

Kids and adults both will love this cooling snack. Run cold water over the cups to make removal easier.

1 (1-lb.) package frozen peach slices,
  partially thawed

2 (8-oz.) cartons blueberry yogurt
2 tablespoons honey, if desired

In a blender or food processor fitted with the metal blade, process peaches, yogurt and honey, if desired, to a puree. Pour into 11 (3-oz.) paper cups or plastic holders, filling each cup about 2/3 full. Freeze 1 hour or until partially frozen. Insert a plastic spoon or a wooden ice cream stick in center of each pop. Freeze 2 hours more or until firm. To serve, peel off paper cup or remove from plastic holders. Makes 11 pops.

**Per pop:
77 calories
0.4 gram fiber**

Cheesy Popcorn

Popcorn is another high-fiber food that is delicious.

2 quarts popped popcorn
1/2 cup (2 oz.) shredded Cheddar cheese

1 teaspoon dried leaf basil
1 teaspoon chili powder

Preheat oven to 300F (150C). In a large bowl, combine popcorn, cheese, basil and chili powder. Pour into a large baking pan. Bake in preheated oven 15 minutes or until cheese melts and popcorn is crisp. Makes 8 cups.

**Per cup:
55 calories
0.3 gram fiber**

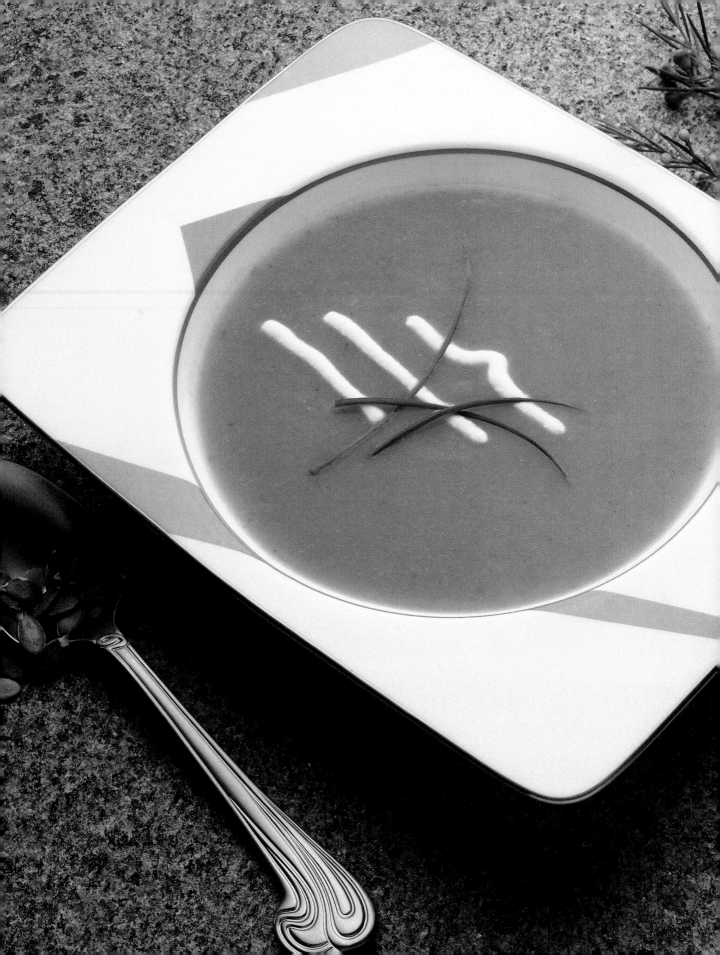

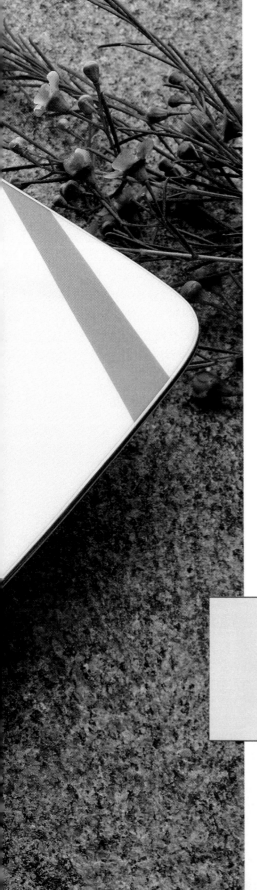

Pumpkin-Apple Soup, page 38

Soups

CHAPTER TWO

Soups

The role of soups can vary from the perfect sandwich accompaniment to the first course of an elegant meal. Soup can even be a main dish. Just as the soup's place on the menu can change, what is called "soup" may vary from a clear broth to a thick puree. A delicious soup can be made by following a recipe completely, or by opening the refrigerator and seeing what fresh vegetables are available.

Some soups, such as Green Split-Pea Soup, page 42, or Hot Beef Borscht, page 37, are best served hot. They are especially welcome on a cold day. Others such as Light Summer Vegetable Soup, page 41, or Pumpkin-Apple Soup, page 38, are excellent served hot or cold. When serving a soup cold, taste for seasoning before serving. Chilling allows time for the flavors to blend and also may decrease the intensity of some seasonings.

As the first course of a meal, soup slows down the pace of eating—it's difficult to eat a hot soup full of crunchy vegetables in a hurry! This allows time for you to relax so your digestive system is better prepared for its job. When serving soup as the first course, select a hearty soup if the rest of the meal is light. However, the soup should be less filling if the remaining dishes are substantial.

Soups are often based on chicken or beef broth so it's necessary to add a word of caution concerning salt or sodium. Canned broths are high in sodium unless you use one of the low-sodium products available. Bouillon cubes are also high in salt, but there are low-sodium versions. If you need to cut down on salt, use one of the low-sodium products that are now in most supermarkets or make your own broth without added salt. Even if you're not cutting down on salt, always taste a soup made with regular commercial broth before adding salt. Otherwise the soup may be too salty.

If you make your own broth, strain and refrigerate it until chilled. Any fat in the broth will float to the top and harden, then it can be easily removed. If you want to use the broth without chilling, use a large spoon or folded paper towel to remove as much of the fat as possible. Homemade broth can be covered and refrigerated up to three days. For longer storage, pour into plastic freezer containers, seal and freeze up to three months.

Hot Beef Borscht

Delicious hot borscht must be the reason beets were created! Vinegar and sugar add a sweet-sour flavor.

1 pound beef stew meat, cut in
   1-inch cubes
5 cups beef broth
5 cups water
1 bay leaf
3 parsley sprigs
2 large carrots, shredded
1 small onion, chopped

2 (1-lb.) cans julienned beets
1/4 small head green cabbage, shredded
1/2 cup red-wine vinegar
2 tablespoons dark-brown sugar
Salt
Freshly ground pepper
1 cup plain low-fat yogurt

In a Dutch oven, combine beef, broth, water, bay leaf and parsley. Bring to a boil. Skim off foam. Reduce heat, cover and simmer 1 hour or until beef is tender. Using a slotted spoon, remove beef, bay leaf and parsley. Discard bay leaf and parsley; cool beef. Add carrots, onion, beets with juice, cabbage, vinegar and brown sugar to cooking liquid. Bring to a boil. Reduce heat, cover and simmer 20 minutes or until vegetables are tender. Season with salt and pepper. Shred beef; return to soup. Heat until hot. Top each serving with yogurt. Makes 8 servings.

**Per serving:
144 calories
1.2 grams fiber**

Beef-Barley Soup

A great soup for a cold winter day!

8 ounces beef stew meat, cut in
   1/2-inch cubes
1 (1 lb.) can crushed Italian-style
   tomatoes
5 cups water
1/3 cup barley
1 large carrot, chopped
1 small onion, chopped

1 large celery stalk, chopped
1 (6-oz.) rutabaga, chopped
1 bay leaf
1/2 teaspoon dried leaf oregano
Hot-pepper sauce
Salt
Freshly ground pepper
1 cup shredded cabbage

In a Dutch oven, combine beef, tomatoes with juice, water, barley, carrot, onion, celery, rutabaga, bay leaf and oregano. Season with hot-pepper sauce, salt and pepper. Bring to a boil. Reduce heat, cover and simmer 40 minutes, stirring occasionally. Add cabbage. Simmer 10 minutes or until cabbage is tender. Makes 6 servings.

**Per serving:
108 calories
1.0 gram fiber**

Shrimp-Pea Soup

Colorful, delicious and easy to prepare!

2 cups fresh green peas or 1 (10-oz.)
   package frozen green peas
8 ounces new red potatoes, cut in
   1/4-inch slices
5 cups chicken broth
1 teaspoon dried leaf tarragon

1 head leaf lettuce, shredded
6 ounces small shrimp, cooked, shelled
Salt
White pepper
Chopped chives

In a medium-size saucepan, combine peas, potatoes, broth and tarragon. Bring to a boil. Reduce heat, cover and simmer 10 minutes or until vegetables are tender. Stir in lettuce. Cover and simmer 5 minutes. Stir in shrimp. Season with salt and white pepper. Heat until hot. Sprinkle each serving with chives. Makes 6 servings.

Pumpkin-Apple Soup

Serve this delicious soup as a first course. (Photo on page 34.)

1 tablespoon butter or margarine
1 tablespoon finely chopped onion
1 large Granny Smith apple, coarsely
   grated or finely chopped
1 cup canned or cooked pumpkin
3 cups chicken broth
1 teaspoon curry powder or to taste

Salt
White pepper
4 tablespoons shelled roasted pumpkin
   seeds, if desired
Plain low-fat yogurt, if desired
Chives, if desired

In a medium-size saucepan, melt butter over medium heat. Add onion. Sauté until softened; do not brown. Add apple, pumpkin, broth and curry powder. Season with salt and white pepper. Bring to a boil. Reduce heat. Cover and simmer, stirring occasionally, 25 minutes or until apple and onion are tender. In a blender or a food processor fitted with the metal blade, process soup in batches to a puree. Reheat if necessary. Sprinkle each serving with pumpkin seeds, if desired. Garnish with piped yogurt and chives, if desired. Makes 4 servings.

Variation
Reduce chicken broth to 2 cups. Follow directions through processing soup to a puree. Pour soup into a medium-size bowl. Stir in 1 cup low-fat milk and 1 additional teaspoon curry powder. Cover and refrigerate until chilled. Serve cold.

Alsatian Onion Soup

This soup from both leeks and onions has a milder onion flavor than regular onion soup. Wash the leeks well under running water to remove all traces of sand.

2 tablespoons butter or margarine
4 cups sliced onions
2 cups sliced leeks, white part only
4 cups chicken broth or 2 cups chicken
  broth and 2 cups beef broth

1 bay leaf
1/4 teaspoon freshly grated nutmeg
Salt
White pepper

In a large saucepan, melt butter over medium heat. Stir in onions and leeks. Reduce heat to low. Cook, stirring occasionally, 15 to 20 minutes or until onions and leeks are very soft. Add broth, bay leaf and nutmeg. Season with salt and white pepper. Cover and simmer 20 minutes. Remove bay leaf. Serve hot. Makes 6 servings.

Per serving:
98 calories
1.2 grams fiber

Eggplant Soup

Greek-style soup with a wonderfully rich flavor and aroma.

1 small eggplant, cut in 1-inch cubes
1 small green bell pepper, chopped
1 medium-size onion, chopped
12 ounces tomatoes, chopped
4 cups beef broth

1 large garlic clove, minced
1 teaspoon dried leaf basil
1 teaspoon dried leaf oregano
Salt
Freshly ground pepper

In a large saucepan, combine eggplant, bell pepper, onion, tomatoes, broth, garlic, basil and oregano. Season with salt and pepper. Bring to a boil. Reduce heat, cover and simmer 30 minutes or until vegetables are tender. Makes 4 servings.

Per serving:
85 calories
2.8 grams fiber

Save the cooking water from vegetables to add to your soups.

Broccoli-Potato Soup

Blue cheese is the unusual ingredient in this soup; it gives a wonderfully rich flavor.

12 ounces broccoli, chopped
12 ounces baking potatoes, peeled, chopped
1 small onion, finely chopped
4 cups chicken broth
Salt

White pepper
2 tablespoons butter or margarine, room temperature
2 tablespoons all-purpose flour
1/2 cup (2 oz.) crumbled blue cheese

Per serving:
276 calories
1.6 grams fiber

In a medium-size saucepan, combine broccoli, potatoes, onion and broth. Season with salt and white pepper. Bring to a boil. Reduce heat. Cover and simmer about 15 minutes or until vegetables are tender. In a blender or food processor fitted with the metal blade, process mixture in batches until vegetables are finely chopped. Return to saucepan. In a small bowl, cream butter and flour to a paste. Stir into soup in small amounts. Cook, stirring constantly, until thickened. Add cheese; cook, stirring constantly, until cheese melts. Makes 4 servings.

Vegetable-Cheese Soup

Rich with Cheddar cheese, this soup has colorful bits of floating vegetables.

6 cups chicken broth
2 large carrots, shredded
2 large celery stalks, finely chopped
1 cup packed chopped spinach
1/4 cup all-purpose flour

2 cups low-fat milk
3/4 cup (3 oz.) shredded Cheddar cheese
1/8 teaspoon freshly grated nutmeg
Salt
White pepper

Per serving:
172 calories
1.1 grams fiber

In a large saucepan, bring broth to a boil. Add carrots, celery and spinach. Bring to a boil again. Reduce heat, cover and simmer 15 minutes or until vegetables are tender. In a small bowl, whisk flour and 1/2 cup of milk until smooth; whisk into hot soup. Whisk in remaining milk. Cook, stirring constantly, 5 minutes or until bubbly and slightly thickened. Stir in cheese until melted. Add nutmeg. Season with salt and white pepper. Makes 4 to 6 servings.

Lentil-Vegetable Soup

Lentils do not need to be soaked before cooking.

1 cup brown lentils	2 large carrots, chopped
3 cups chicken broth	1 small onion, chopped
2 parsley sprigs	1 small garlic clove, minced
1 bay leaf	1 teaspoon dried leaf thyme
1 teaspoon olive oil	Hot-pepper sauce
12 ounces tomatoes, chopped	Salt
2 large celery stalks, chopped	Freshly ground pepper

In a large saucepan, combine lentils, broth, parsley, bay leaf and olive oil. Bring to a boil. Stir in tomatoes, celery, carrots, onion, garlic and thyme. Season with hot-pepper sauce, salt and pepper. Bring to a boil. Reduce heat. Cover and simmer, stirring occasionally, 45 minutes or until lentils and vegetables are tender. Remove bay leaf and parsley. Makes 4 servings.

> **Per serving:**
> 195 calories
> 3.1 grams fiber

Light Summer Vegetable Soup

Serve this delicious soup hot or chilled.

1 tablespoon olive oil	1 pound tomatoes, chopped
1 small onion, chopped	2 large zucchini, chopped
2 cups chicken broth	6 ounces mushrooms, sliced
1 cup water	1/2 teaspoon dried leaf oregano
2 medium-size ears of corn, kernels cut off cob or 1 (12-oz.) can whole-kernel corn	Hot-pepper sauce
	Salt
	Freshly ground pepper

In a medium-size saucepan, heat olive oil over medium heat. Add onion; sauté until softened. Add broth, water, corn and tomatoes. Bring to a boil. Reduce heat, cover and simmer 10 minutes. Stir in zucchini, mushrooms and oregano. Season with hot-pepper sauce, salt and pepper. Cover and simmer 20 minutes or until vegetables are tender. Makes 6 servings.

> **Per serving:**
> 103 calories
> 1.9 grams fiber

Quick Double-Corn Chowder

This is an adaptation of an early American dish. There are two types of corn, which is a good source of fiber, in this easy recipe.

2 tablespoons butter or margarine
1 small onion, chopped
1 medium-size zucchini, shredded
1 tablespoon finely chopped fresh
   parsley
1 (1-lb.) can cream-style corn

1 (12-oz.) can whole-kernel corn,
   drained
2 cups low-fat milk
Hot-pepper sauce
Salt
White pepper

Per serving:
155 calories
2.4 grams fiber

In a medium-size saucepan, melt butter over medium heat. Add onion, zucchini and parsley. Cook until onion is tender. Stir in cream-style corn, whole-kernel corn and milk. Season with hot-pepper sauce, salt and white pepper. Reduce heat. Uncover and simmer 10 minutes; do not boil. Makes 4 to 6 servings.

Green Split-Pea Soup

With cold wind howling at the door, what soup could be more welcome?

1 pound green split peas
2 quarts water
1 bay leaf
1 teaspoon vegetable oil
1 cup chopped lean ham

1 small onion, chopped
1 medium-size carrot, diced
1 large garlic clove, minced
Salt

Per serving:
290 calories
1.1 grams fiber

In a large saucepan, combine peas, water, bay leaf and oil. Bring to a boil, stirring occasionally. Boil 10 minutes. Reduce heat, cover and simmer 40 minutes, stirring occasionally. Add ham, onion, carrot and garlic. Season with salt. Cover; simmer 30 minutes or until peas and vegetables are tender. Remove bay leaf. Makes 6 servings.

Wild-Rice Soup

There are many versions of this soup. I particularly like the contrast between the rice and the spinach.

5 cups chicken broth
1/2 cup wild rice
1 small onion, diced
2 medium-size carrots, diced
1/2 bunch spinach, shredded

4 ounces mushrooms, chopped
Salt
Freshly ground pepper
2 tablespoons dry sherry

In a large saucepan, combine broth, rice, onion and carrots. Bring to a boil. Reduce heat, cover and simmer 35 minutes, stirring occasionally. Stir in spinach and mushrooms. Season with salt and pepper. Cook 5 minutes or until rice and vegetables are tender. Stir in sherry. Makes 4 servings.

Per serving:
173 calories
2.5 grams fiber

Commercially prepared chicken and beef broth and bouillon cubes are high in salt. However, there are low-sodium versions available. Look for these or make your own unsalted stocks.

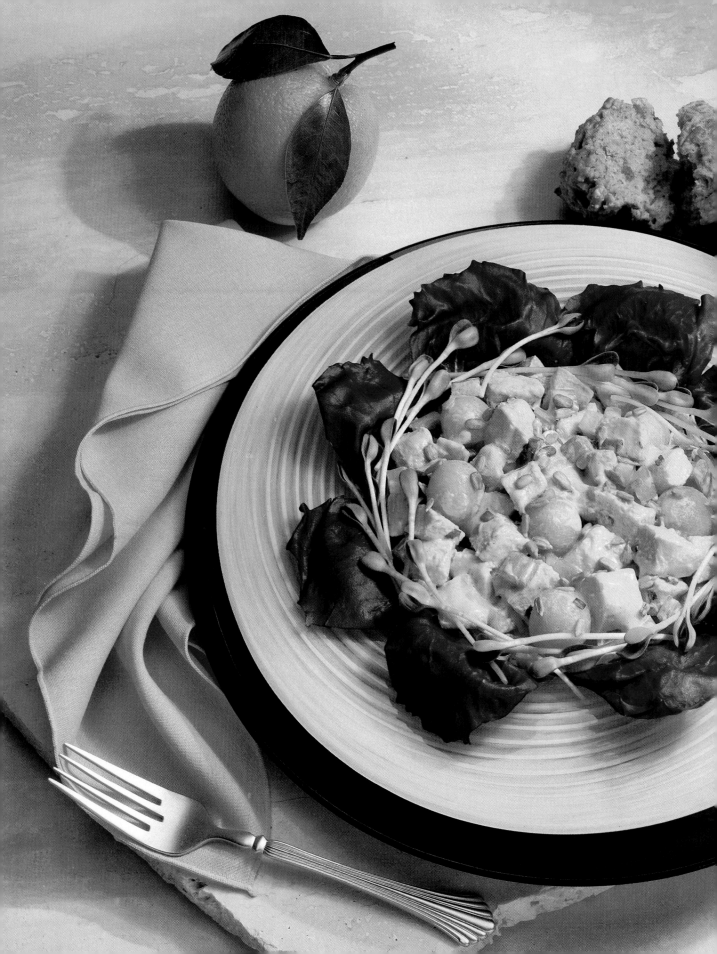

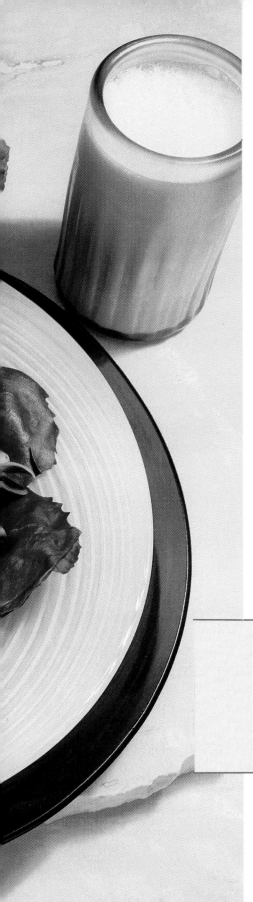

Banana-Marmalade Muffins, page 124; Chicken-Melon Salad, page 57

Salads

CHAPTER THREE

Salads

Like soups, salads play many roles. They can be served as tempting appetizers to perk up appetites or as side dishes to offer new textures and flavors to complement the main dish. They can be a palate cleanser after the main dish, or a salad can be the main dish, especially for a summer luncheon or light supper.

Because salads are made mostly of raw vegetables and fruits, they are excellent sources of both soluble and insoluble fiber. Other salad components, such as nuts, grains and dried bean also contribute fiber.

When selecting greens for salad, look for greens that are crisp and fresh. Wash and thoroughly dry greens before combining with other ingredients. Wet or damp greens will dilute the salad dressing. If the salad is composed mostly of greens, toss with a small amount of dressing just before serving to prevent the salad from being limp.

Fresh herbs can be used in salads to good advantage. If fresh herbs are not available, used dried herbs or herb-flavored vinegars.

Vinegars used for salads include red-wine vinegar, white-wine vinegar, balsamic vinegar, fruit-flavored vinegar and rice vinegar. The wine vinegars can be used interchangeably, but don't use the red-wine vinegar when a light color is important to the final appearance of the salad. Balsamic vinegar is a strong, dark vinegar with an aromatic flavor; it is usually used in small amounts. Several fruit-flavored vinegars are available, such as raspberry-flavored vinegar. Rice vinegar is a mild-flavored vinegar made from rice; it is available plain or lightly seasoned with sugar. Lemon juice or lime juice is also used to add tanginess to a salad instead of vinegar.

Oils used for salads are usually mild in flavor. Occasionally a special oil, such as hazelnut oil or walnut oil, is added in a small amount for flavor. Olive oil is a popular choice for salads; choose virgin olive oil or oil from the first pressing. Because oil has about 125 calories per tablespoon, it is important to limit its use if a low-calorie dressing is desired. Several recipes use yogurt as the base for low-calorie creamy dressing.

Double-Tangerine &
Cranberry Mold

Two winter treats, tangerines and cranberries, are combined in this salad. There's no need to add sugar; the natural sweetness of the concentrated juice is enough.

2 tablespoons unflavored gelatin powder
1/2 cup water
1 (12-oz.) can frozen tangerine-juice
   concentrate, thawed
3 medium-size tangerines

1 (12-oz.) package cranberries
2 large celery stalks, finely chopped
1/2 cup chopped pecans
3 to 4 leaf-lettuce leaves

Per serving:
145 calories
1.9 grams fiber

Lightly spray a 4-cup mold with nonstick cooking spray. In a small saucepan, combine gelatin and water. Let stand 5 minutes or until softened. Cook, stirring constantly, over medium heat until gelatin dissolves. In a medium-size bowl, combine gelatin mixture with tangerine juice. Let stand until slightly thickened. Thinly slice tangerines crosswise; remove seeds. Cut slices in half. Discard any spoiled cranberries. In a food processor fitted with the metal blade, process 1/2 of tangerines and 1/2 of cranberries until finely chopped. Repeat with remaining tangerines and cranberries. Stir chopped tangerines and cranberries into thickened gelatin mixture. Pour into prepared mold. Cover and refrigerate 3 to 4 hours or until completely set. To serve, place lettuce leaves on a serving plate. Run a knife around edge of mold to loosen. Invert mold on lettuce-lined plate. Wet a dish towel with hot water; wring dry. Wrap hot towel around mold a few seconds. Remove towel and mold. Makes 6 servings.

Variation
Substitute 1 large orange and 1 (12-oz.) can frozen orange-juice concentrate for tangerines and frozen tangerine-juice concentrate.

Tropical Fruit Salad

An excellent way to serve the exotic caramabola or star fruit when it's in season. (Photo on cover.)

2 large bananas, if desired
1 tablespoon lemon juice
2 kiwifruits, peeled, cut crosswise in 1/4-inch slices
1 (15-1/4-oz.) can pineapple slices (juice pack), drained, cut in halves, or fresh pineapple

1 pint strawberries
1 papaya, if desired, cut in quarters
1 caramabola, if desired, sliced crosswise in 1/4-inch slices
1/4 cup papaya nectar
2 teaspoons honey
1/2 cup plain low-fat yogurt

If using bananas, peel and cut in half crosswise, then cut each half lengthwise. In a medium-size bowl, gently toss bananas with lemon juice. Arrange fruits on a large platter. To make dressing, in a small bowl, stir nectar and honey until honey dissolves; mix in yogurt. Pour dressing over salad. Makes 6 servings.

Variation

For a thicker dressing, substitute pureed papaya for papaya nectar.

Melon Cup

Use a melon baller to make perfectly round balls, or cut melons in cubes. One-fourth of a large cantaloupe yields about one cup of balls.

1 cup watermelon balls
1 cup cantaloupe balls
1 cup honeydew balls

2 tablespoons orange-flavored liqueur or thawed frozen orange-juice concentrate

In a glass serving dish, combine melon balls. Drizzle with liqueur. Cover and refrigerate until chilled. To serve, stir gently. Makes 4 to 6 servings.

Orange & Beet Salad

Arrange this attractive salad on individual, lettuce-lined salad plates, if desired.

3 medium-size oranges
1/2 cup plain low-fat yogurt
3/4 teaspoon prepared horseradish
Salt

Freshly ground pepper
1 (1-lb.) can julienne beets,
   well drained

Grate 1 teaspoon peel from 1 orange; set aside. Hold oranges over a medium-size bowl to catch juice while peeling and slicing. Peel oranges, removing all bitter white pith. Cut oranges crosswise in 1/4-inch slices; set aside. In a medium-size bowl, combine reserved orange peel, 1 tablespoon of reserved orange juice, yogurt and horseradish. Season with salt and pepper. Stir in beets. Cover and refrigerate orange slices and beets separately about 30 minutes or until chilled. To serve, mound beets in center of a serving plate. Overlap orange slices around beets. Makes 6 servings.

Per serving:
62 calories
0.8 gram fiber

Citrus Salad

Avocados and coconut are high in fat, so use them only occasionally if you're watching calories.

2 medium-size pink grapefruit
4 large oranges
1 medium-size avocado

1/2 cup pomegranate seeds
2 tablespoons dry sherry
1 teaspoon sugar

Peel grapefruit and oranges, removing all bitter white pith. Holding fruit over a medium-size bowl to collect juices, cut between membranes in sections. Squeeze membranes to extract all juice; set aside. Alternate grapefruit and orange sections on 6 salad plates, forming a ring. Set aside. Slice avocado in half; discard seed. Using a small melon baller, cut avocado in balls. Toss balls in reserved juice to prevent browning. Arrange 3 to 5 balls in center of each salad. Sprinkle with pomegranate seeds. To make dressing, in a small bowl, combine 2 tablespoons of reserved juice, sherry and sugar. Stir until sugar dissolves. Drizzle dressing over salad. Makes 6 servings.

Per serving:
170 calories
2.6 grams fiber

Orange-Onion Salad

A good choice for a winter salad when the orange crop is at its peak.

1/2 head red-leaf lettuce, torn in
    bite-size pieces
1/2 bunch spinach, trimmed, torn in
    bite-size pieces
1 large orange, peeled, sectioned
1/2 medium-size red onion, cut in thin
    slices, separated in rings

2 tablespoons thawed frozen
    orange-juice concentrate
1 tablespoon vegetable oil
1 tablespoon white-wine vinegar
Salt
Freshly ground pepper

In a serving bowl, combine lettuce, spinach, orange and onion. To make dressing, in a small bowl, whisk orange-juice concentrate, oil and vinegar until combined. Season with salt and pepper. Pour dressing over salad; toss to combine. Makes 4 servings.

Orange, Green & White Salad

Serve in a divided dish for a colorful presentation.

1 large carrot, shredded
2 medium-size turnips, shredded
1 medium-size zucchini, shredded
3 tablespoons olive oil
3 tablespoons seasoned rice vinegar
1 teaspoon dried leaf tarragon or basil

Salt
Freshly ground pepper
1 tomato rose, if desired
Cilantro sprig, if desired
2 strips lemon peel, if desired

Place carrot, turnips and zucchini in 3 separate medium-size bowls; set aside. To make dressing, in a small bowl, whisk olive oil, vinegar and tarragon until slightly thickened. Season with salt and pepper. Pour 1/3 of dressing over each vegetable; toss to combine. Cover and refrigerate each salad 1 hour. Toss again. Drain salads; discard dressing. Arrange salads separately in a serving dish. Garnish with tomato rose, cilantro and lemon peel, if desired. Makes 6 servings.

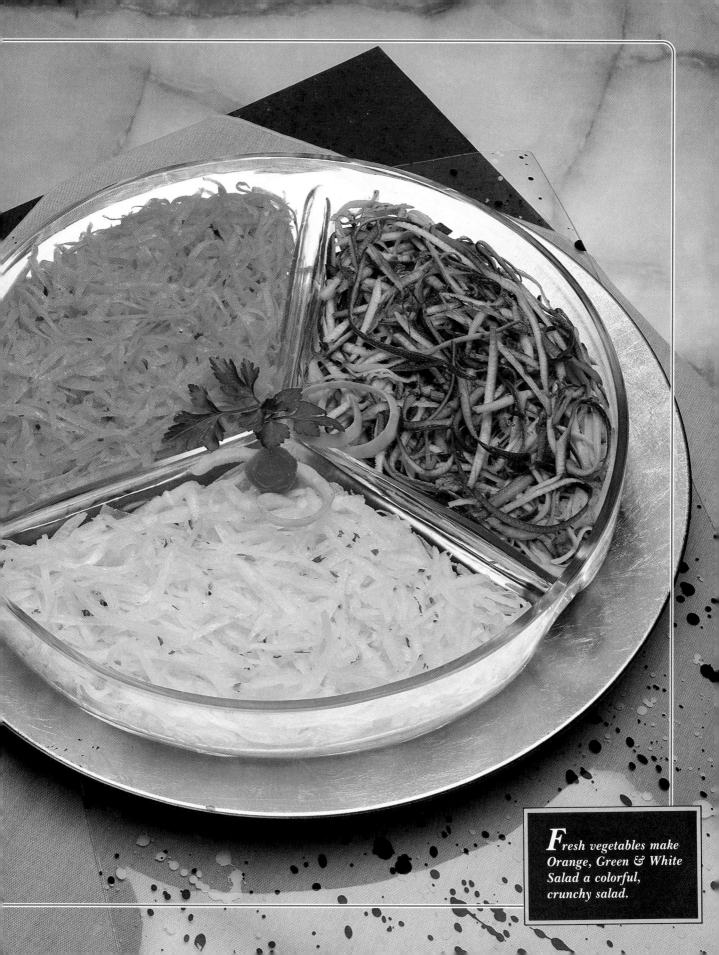

*F*resh vegetables make
Orange, Green & White
Salad a colorful,
crunchy salad.

"Green" Salad

Make this crunchy salad up to 8 hours ahead.

1 (10-oz.) package frozen green peas, thawed, drained
2 large celery stalks, chopped
1 medium-size green bell pepper, cubed
1 small cucumber, peeled, cubed
4 green onions, chopped
1/4 cup mayonnaise
1/4 cup plain low-fat yogurt

1 tablespoon Dijon-style mustard
1 tablespoon lemon juice
1 teaspoon dried dill weed or dried leaf tarragon
Salt
White pepper
About 6 large leaf-lettuce leaves

In a medium-size bowl, combine peas, celery, bell pepper, cucumber and onions. Set aside. To make dressing, in a small bowl, combine mayonnaise, yogurt, mustard, lemon juice and dill. Season with salt and white pepper. Pour dressing over vegetable mixture; toss to combine. Cover and refrigerate about 1 hour. Arrange lettuce leaves around edge of a serving bowl. Spoon salad into center. Makes 6 servings.

Cucumber-Yogurt Salad

There are many variations of this classic dish. It's delicious with grilled meats or Eggplant Casserole, page 64.

1 large cucumber, thinly sliced
1 small red onion, thinly sliced
2 large stalks celery, thinly sliced
1 garlic clove, minced

1/2 teaspoon ground cumin
Salt
White pepper
1/2 cup plain low-fat yogurt

Pat cucumber slices with paper towels to remove some moisture. In a medium-size bowl, combine cucumber, onion, celery, garlic and cumin. Season with salt and white pepper. Gently stir in yogurt. Cover and refrigerate until chilled. Makes 4 servings.

Variation
Substitute 1 tablespoon chopped fresh dill or 1 teaspoon dried dill weed for cumin.

Potato Salad

Yogurt adds a nice tanginess to the dressing without a lot of calories!

1 pound red potatoes
2 large celery stalks, chopped
1 small onion, chopped
2 tablespoons chopped chives or
   green onion tops
2 small sweet pickles, chopped
1/3 cup mayonnaise

1/3 cup low-fat plain yogurt
1 teaspoon Dijon-style mustard
1 teaspoon dried dill weed
Salt
Freshly ground pepper
1 hard-cooked egg
1 sweet pickle, if desired

In a large saucepan, cook potatoes in boiling salted water about 25 minutes or until fork-tender. Drain and cool. Cut unpeeled potatoes in 1-1/2-inch cubes. In a medium-size bowl, combine potatoes, celery, onion, chives and chopped pickles. Set aside. To make dressing, in a small bowl, combine mayonnaise, yogurt, mustard and dill. Season with salt and pepper. Pour dressing over potato mixture; toss gently until combined. Cover and refrigerate until chilled or up to 2 days. To serve, slice hard-cooked egg. Arrange egg slices around edge of salad. If desired, cut sweet pickle in a fan; place in center of salad. Makes 4 servings.

**Per serving:
300 calories
2.6 grams fiber**

Tomato & Artichoke-Heart Salad

Great for last-minute guests because it takes only minutes to prepare. It's especially good with fresh basil.

1 (6-oz.) jar marinated artichoke hearts
4 (4-oz.) tomatoes, cut crosswise in slices
1 tablespoon chopped fresh basil or
   1 teaspoon dried leaf basil

Salt
Freshly ground pepper
1 tablespoon balsamic vinegar or
   white-wine vinegar

Drain artichoke hearts well; reserve marinade. Cut artichoke hearts in quarters. Arrange tomatoes in center of 4 salad plates. Place artichoke-heart quarters around tomatoes. Sprinkle with basil. Season with salt and pepper. To make dressing, in a small bowl, whisk 2 tablespoons reserved marinade and vinegar until thickened. Drizzle dressing over tomatoes. Makes 4 servings.

**Per serving:
98 calories
2.6 grams fiber**

Fennel Salad

Fennel has a slight anise flavor and a texture similar to celery.

1 large fennel bulb, cut crosswise in 1/4-inch slices
2 large Red Delicious apples, chopped, tossed with lemon juice
1/2 cup diced Swiss cheese (about 2 oz.)

2 tablespoons plain low-fat yogurt
1 tablespoon olive oil
1 tablespoon white-wine vinegar
1 teaspoon Dijon-style mustard

Per serving:
157 calories
2.6 grams fiber

In a medium-size bowl, combine fennel, apples and cheese. To make dressing, in a small bowl, whisk yogurt, olive oil, vinegar and mustard. Pour dressing over salad; toss to combine. Makes 4 servings.

Carrot Salad

Instead of the usual mayonnaise-type dressing, this salad is tossed with a light oil-and-vinegar dressing. (Photo on page 60.)

3 large carrots, shredded
2 medium-size oranges, peeled, sectioned
1 medium-size Red Delicious apple, chopped

2 tablespoons vegetable oil
3 tablespoons raspberry-flavored vinegar or white-wine vinegar
1 teaspoon sugar
1/4 cup pecans, chopped

Per serving:
141 calories
1.8 grams fiber

In a serving bowl, combine carrots, oranges and apple. To make dressing, in a small bowl, whisk oil, vinegar and sugar until sugar dissolves. Pour dressing over salad; toss to combine. Sprinkle with pecans. Makes 4 to 6 servings.

Southwestern Gazpacho Salad

A take-off on gazpacho, Southwestern Gazpacho Salad is a colorful and delicious addition to a Southwestern-style buffet.

1 large green bell pepper, coarsely chopped
1 small cucumber, peeled, coarsely chopped
1 small onion, coarsely chopped
1 pound tomatoes, coarsely chopped

1 (4-oz.) can diced chilies, drained
2 tablespoons minced fresh cilantro
2 tablespoons seasoned rice vinegar
2 tablespoons vegetable oil
Freshly ground pepper
Salt

In a medium-size bowl, combine bell pepper, cucumber, onion, tomatoes, chilies, cilantro, vinegar and oil. Season with pepper. Cover and refrigerate about 4 hours, stirring occasionally. Season with salt. Drain, if necessary. Makes 6 servings.

Per serving:
69 calories
1.1 grams fiber

Marinated Vegetables

Perfect for a picnic when packed into a tightly sealed container.

1/2 small head cauliflower, separated in flowerets
2 medium-size carrots, cut diagonally in 1/4-inch-thick slices
1 large celery stalk, cut diagonally in 1/4-inch-thick slices

1 medium-size cucumber, scored lengthwise, sliced
1 medium-size tomato, cut in 8 wedges

Honey-Sesame Dressing:
1/4 cup chicken broth
2 tablespoons vegetable oil
2 tablespoons white-wine vinegar
1 tablespoon honey

1 teaspoon sesame oil
Salt
Freshly ground pepper

In a large saucepan, steam cauliflower, carrots and celery over boiling water 4 minutes or until crisp-tender. Rinse with cold water; cool. In a large bowl, combine cauliflower, carrots, celery, cucumber and tomato. Prepare dressing. Pour over salad; toss to combine. Cover and refrigerate 2 hours, gently tossing vegetables in dressing occasionally. Drain salad; discard dressing. Makes 4 to 6 servings.

Per serving:
137 calories
1.8 grams fiber

Honey-Sesame Dressing:
In a small bowl, whisk broth, oil, vinegar, honey and sesame oil until combined. Season with salt and pepper.

Garden Salad

Seasoned rice vinegar adds a delightful sweet-sour taste.

1 head leaf lettuce, torn in
   bite-size pieces
1 large green bell pepper, cut in
   1/4-inch strips
2 large carrots, cut in thin
   diagonal slices

1 large tomato, chopped
2 tablespoons seasoned rice vinegar
2 tablespoons olive oil
Salt
Freshly ground pepper

In a salad bowl, combine lettuce, bell pepper, carrots and tomato. To make dressing, in a small bowl, whisk vinegar and olive oil until slightly thickened. Pour dressing over salad; toss to combine. Season with salt and pepper. Toss again. Makes 4 to 6 servings.

Mushroom Salad

Sun-dried tomatoes add a nice color and flavor, but can be omitted if not available.

4 ounces mushrooms, sliced
1 ounce sun-dried tomatoes, rinsed,
   chopped
1/4 cup (1 oz.) shredded skim-milk
   mozzarella cheese
1/2 teaspoon dried leaf basil
1 tablespoon raspberry-flavored vinegar

1 tablespoon fresh lime juice
1/4 cup olive oil
Salt
Freshly ground pepper
1 bunch spinach, trimmed, torn in
   bite-size pieces

In a medium-size bowl, combine mushrooms, tomatoes, cheese and basil. Set aside. To make dressing, in a small bowl, whisk vinegar, lime juice and olive oil until slightly thickened. Season with salt and pepper. Add 3 tablespoons of dressing to mushroom mixture; toss to combine. Let stand at room temperature 15 minutes. Arrange spinach on 4 salad plates. Spoon mushroom mixture over spinach. Drizzle with remaining dressing. Makes 4 servings.

Chicken-Melon Salad

A wonderful summer luncheon salad. Serve with Whole-Wheat Potato Rolls, page 118, or your favorite muffins. (Photo on page 44.)

12 ounces cooked chicken, cut in 1-inch chunks (about 3 cups)
2 cups cantaloupe balls
2 large celery stalks, chopped
3 green onions, finely chopped
Salt

Freshly ground pepper
1 small bunch radicchio
1 (4-oz.) carton sunflower sprouts or alfalfa sprouts
4 teaspoons sunflower kernels

Chutney Dressing:
2 tablespoons mango chutney, chopped
3/4 cup plain low-fat yogurt
1/4 cup mayonnaise

1 tablespoon honey mustard
1 teaspoon curry powder

Prepare dressing; set aside. In a medium-size bowl, combine chicken, cantaloupe, celery and onions. Stir dressing into chicken mixture. Season with salt and pepper. Cover and refrigerate 30 minutes. Arrange radicchio around edges of 4 plates. Spread sprouts in center of plates. Mound salad in center of sprouts. Sprinkle with sunflower kernels. Makes 4 servings.

Per serving:
384 calories
1.7 grams fiber

Chutney Dressing:
In a small bowl, combine chutney, yogurt, mayonnaise, honey mustard and curry powder.

Turkey-Cranberry Salad

Don't wait until Thanksgiving to prepare this delicious combination! Serve on fresh spinach for an attractive presentation.

1-1/2 pounds cooked turkey, cut in 1-inch cubes (about 6 cups)
4 ounces bean sprouts
1 small Granny Smith apple, finely chopped
2 large celery stalks, chopped
4 green onions, chopped

Salt
Freshly ground pepper
1/4 cup mayonnaise
1/2 cup plain low-fat yogurt
1 tablespoon lemon juice
1 (1-lb.) can whole-berry cranberry sauce, drained

In a large bowl, combine turkey, bean sprouts, apple, celery and onions. Season with salt and pepper. To make dressing, in a small bowl, combine mayonnaise, yogurt and lemon juice. Stir in cranberry sauce. Gently combine dressing and turkey mixture. Makes 6 servings.

Per serving:
306 calories
0.8 gram fiber

Tabbouleh

Use boiling water to rehydrate bulgur more quickly. Reduce lemon juice slightly if you prefer a less tangy flavor.

1-1/2 cups bulgur (7 to 8 oz.)
3 cups boiling water
1 cup minced fresh parsley
8 ounces tomatoes, finely chopped
4 green onions, minced

2 tablespoons minced fresh mint leaves
1/4 cup plus 2 tablespoons lemon juice
2 tablespoons olive oil
Salt
Freshly ground pepper

In a medium-size bowl, combine bulgur and water. Cover; let stand about 1 hour or until water is absorbed and bulgur is tender. Squeeze out excess moisture. In a serving bowl, combine bulgur, parsley, tomatoes, green onions and mint. To make dressing, in a small bowl, whisk lemon juice and olive oil until combined. Pour dressing over salad; toss to combine. Season with salt and pepper. Cover and refrigerate until chilled. Makes 8 servings.

Brown-Rice Salad

Rice and beans complement each other making this a balanced-protein dish.

1-1/2 cups Basic Brown Rice, page 103, cooled
1 (15-oz.) can red kidney beans, drained, rinsed
1 (8-oz.) can whole-kernel corn, drained
1 large celery stalk, chopped

6 green onions, finely chopped
2 tablespoons chopped fresh parsley
1/4 cup olive oil
2 tablespoons tarragon-flavored vinegar
Salt
Freshly ground pepper

In a medium-size bowl, combine rice, beans, corn, celery, onions and parsley. To make dressing, in a small bowl, whisk olive oil and vinegar until slightly thickened. Pour dressing over rice mixture; toss to combine. Season with salt and pepper. Makes 6 servings.

White-Bean Salad

Rinsed canned white beans can be used in this salad. Serve as an entree or as a side dish.

3-1/2 cups cooked white beans, Basic
    Beans, page 102
2 tablespoons olive oil
2 tablespoons seasoned rice vinegar
1 tablespoon white-wine vinegar

1 large tomato, chopped
1/2 large green bell pepper, chopped
1 large celery stalk, chopped
Salt
White pepper

In a medium-size bowl, combine beans, olive oil and vinegars. Stir in tomato, bell pepper and celery. Season with salt and white pepper. Makes 4 servings.

**Per serving:
261 calories
3.1 grams fiber**

Yogurt-Orange Dressing

Serve with fresh fruit.

1/4 cup thawed frozen orange-juice
    concentrate

1 cup low-fat plain yogurt

In a small bowl, combine orange-juice concentrate and yogurt until blended. Do not overmix or dressing will be thin. Makes about 1-1/4 cups.

**Per tablespoon:
13 calories
0.0 gram fiber**

Light Blue Cheese Dressing

Serve with assorted salad greens.

1 cup plain low-fat yogurt
1 teaspoon honey

1/4 cup (2 oz.) crumbled blue cheese

In a blender or a food processor fitted with the metal blade, process yogurt, honey and blue cheese just until blended. Makes about 1 cup.

**Per tablespoon:
17 calories
0.0 gram fiber**

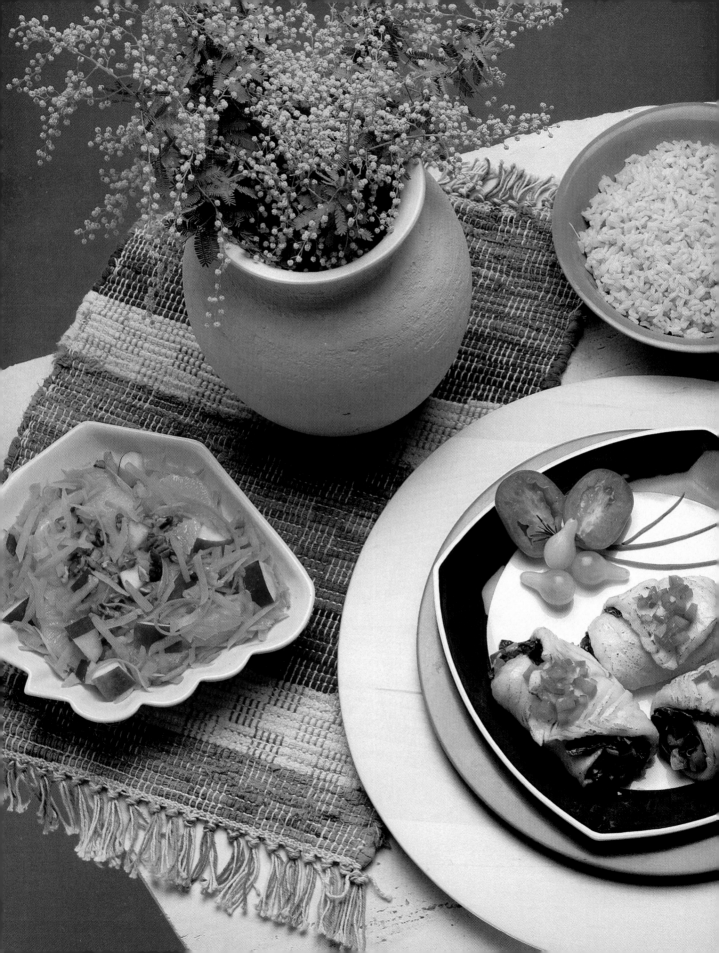

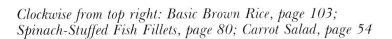

Clockwise from top right: Basic Brown Rice, page 103; Spinach-Stuffed Fish Fillets, page 80; Carrot Salad, page 54

Main Dishes

CHAPTER FOUR

Main Dishes

Meat by itself contains no fiber, because fiber comes from plants. So the meats, chicken and fish in this chapter have been combined with vegetables to make stews, casseroles and other dishes. For example, chicken is cooked with bell peppers and carrots in a delicious mustard sauce, and red snapper is stuffed with a spinach and tomato mixture, then grilled. Chicken Primavera, page 72, is a colorful mixture of vegetables, chicken and pasta. Many of the dishes need only a green salad and a whole-grain bread or brown rice to make a complete meal.

The skin has been removed from the chicken and turkey and meats were well trimmed to reduce the amount of fat in the recipes. If using ground beef, use the leanest that is available in your market. If you don't know which one to choose, ask the butcher what percentage of fat is in each type. Regular ground beef may contain about 30 percent fat. The leanest type is usually 10 percent fat.

In the case of fish, the fatty fishes, such as salmon and tuna, may be better! Recent research has shown that the omega-3 fatty acids from fish may be protective against heart disease. This is one of the reasons that experts suggest that we increase our intake of fish and seafood. If fresh fish is not available in your area, try to find a source of good frozen fish. Frozen fish that has been processed correctly and kept frozen may be a better choice than less-than-fresh fish. Check package for frost and signs of thawing before buying. Cook fish just until it turns from translucent to opaque. Check by probing with a fork in the thickest part.

Serving sizes are based on four ounces of uncooked meat per person.

Beef Rouladen

This recipe is adapted from the wonderful rouladen my German landlady, Frau Neufang, used to make.

6 (4-oz.) beef round tip steaks, pounded
   1/4-inch thick
2 large carrots, cut in 1/4-inch strips
2 celery stalks, cut in 1/4-inch strips
1 medium-size onion, thinly sliced
About 1-1/2 teaspoons dried leaf thyme
Salt
Freshly ground pepper
1/4 cup whole-wheat flour

2 tablespoons vegetable oil
1 large garlic clove, minced
1-1/2 cups beef broth
1/2 cup dry red wine
2 bay leaves
1-1/2 tablespoons all-purpose flour
Cold water
Chopped fresh parsley

Place steaks on a flat surface. Arrange 4 carrots strips, 4 celery strips and a few onion slices on end of 1 steak. Season steak with thyme, salt and pepper. Roll up steak jelly-roll style. Secure steak roll with a wooden pick. Trim off vegetables even with steak; reserve trimmed vegetables. Repeat with remaining steaks. Lightly coat rolls with whole-wheat flour. In a 10-inch skillet, heat oil over medium heat. Add floured rolls; cook until lightly browned on all sides. Add remaining vegetables, garlic, broth, wine and bay leaves. Bring to a boil. Reduce heat, cover and simmer 1-1/2 hours or until beef is fork-tender. Place rolls in a serving dish; discard bay leaves. In a small bowl, make a paste with all-purpose flour and a little cold water. Stir into cooking liquid. Bring to a boil. Cook, stirring constantly, until thickened. Taste for seasoning; pour over rolls. Sprinkle with parsley. Makes 6 servings.

Per serving:
272 calories
1.5 grams fiber

Veggie Meat Loaf

Make a really great sandwich with leftover meat loaf.

1 medium-size zucchini, grated
1 medium-size carrot, grated
1 medium-size onion, finely chopped
1 cup regular rolled oats
1 egg
1 pound extra-lean ground beef

1 pound turkey sausage
1/4 teaspoon hot-pepper sauce
1 teaspoon salt
1/4 cup water
Tomato Sauce, Spinach Fritata, page
   134, if desired

Preheat oven to 350F (175C). In a medium-size bowl, combine zucchini, carrot, onion, oats, egg, beef, sausage, hot-pepper sauce, salt and water until thoroughly mixed. Lightly pack mixture into a 9" x 5" loaf pan. Bake in preheated oven 1-1/4 hours or until meat loaf is firm in center and pulls away from sides of pan; center of meat loaf should reach 170F (75 C). Spoon off fat that accumulates during baking. Let stand 5 to 10 minutes to firm before slicing. Serve with Tomato Sauce, if desired. Makes 10 servings.

Eggplant Casserole

Cinnamon gives a true Middle-Eastern flavor. I always broil eggplant slices rather than frying—this saves a lot of calories!

8 ounces lean ground beef
1 medium-size onion, chopped
2 large garlic cloves, minced
1 (28-oz.) can crushed Italian-style
   tomatoes
3/4 cup dry red wine
2 tablespoons chopped fresh basil or 2
   teaspoons dried leaf basil
1 tablespoon chopped fresh thyme or 1
   teaspoon dried leaf thyme
Dash ground cinnamon

Salt
Freshly ground pepper
1 (1-1/4-lb.) eggplant, peeled, cut
   lengthwise in 1/4-inch-thick slices
8 ounces part-skim mozzarella cheese,
   thinly sliced
3/4 cup fresh whole-wheat bread crumbs
2 tablespoons wheat germ
1 tablespoon unprocessed wheat bran
2 tablespoons grated Parmesan cheese

In a large saucepan, cook beef without added fat over medium heat until no longer pink, stirring to break up meat. Remove with a slotted spoon. Add onion and garlic to fat remaining in pan; cook until onion is softened. Drain off any excess fat. Return beef to pan. Stir in tomatoes, wine, basil, thyme and cinnamon. Season with salt and pepper. Simmer over low heat 20 minutes or until mixture thickens. Meanwhile, position oven rack about 4 inches from heat source; preheat broiler. Arrange eggplant on a nonstick baking sheet. Broil in preheated broiler about 5 minutes or until fork-tender. Preheat oven to 350F (175C). Grease a shallow 2-1/2-quart casserole dish. Arrange 1/2 of eggplant slices in bottom of greased dish; top with 1/2 of tomato mixture. Spread 1/2 of mozzarella cheese over tomato mixture. Repeat with remaining eggplant, tomato mixture and mozzarella cheese. In a small bowl, combine bread crumbs, wheat germ, wheat bran and Parmesan cheese. Sprinkle over casserole. Bake in preheated oven 30 minutes or until hot and bubbly and topping is browned. Let stand 10 minutes before serving. Makes 6 servings.

Stuffed Cabbage

Both tasty and nutritious, this is one of my favorites.

2/3 cup bulgur	Salt
1-1/4 cups boiling water	Freshly ground pepper
1 (2-lb.) head green cabbage	1 (28-oz.) can crushed Italian-style
8 ounces lean ground beef	tomatoes
1 small onion, chopped	1/2 cup chicken broth
1 large garlic clove, minced	1/2 cup dry red wine
1-1/2 teaspoons caraway seeds, crushed	1 teaspoon dried leaf thyme
Hot-pepper sauce	2 bay leaves

In a small bowl, combine bulgur and boiling water. Let stand 30 minutes. Remove any damaged leaves from outside of cabbage. Cut about 1/2 inch off bottom of cabbage to release ends of outer leaves. In a large saucepan, blanch cabbage 10 to 15 minutes or until leaves loosen. Outer leaves can be removed as they loosen. Drain cabbage; cool. In a medium-size skillet, brown beef without added fat over medium-high heat, stirring to break up meat. Add onions and garlic. Cook, stirring occasionally, until onions are softened. Drain off any excess fat. Add caraway seeds. Season with hot-pepper sauce, salt and pepper. Stir in 1 cup of tomatoes; set aside. Separate 8 to 10 large outer leaves from cabbage; set aside. Finely chop remaining cabbage; stir into meat mixture. Drain bulgur, if necessary; stir into meat mixture. Preheat oven to 375F (190C). Grease a shallow 3-quart baking dish. Place cabbage leaves on a flat surface. Spoon about 1/3 cup meat mixture near stem end of each cabbage leaf. Fold sides over mixture and roll, starting at stem end. Place cabbage rolls in greased dish; set aside. In a medium-size bowl, combine remaining tomatoes, broth, wine and thyme. Pour over cabbage rolls. Add bay leaves. Cover with a lid or foil. Bake in preheated oven about 40 minutes or until cabbage is tender. Discard bay leaves. Makes 4 to 6 servings.

Per serving:
302 calories
2.2 grams fiber

Easy Chili

A delicious, nontraditional version!

8 ounces lean ground beef
1 large onion, chopped
1 large garlic clove, minced
1 (28-oz.) can crushed Italian-style
    tomatoes
2 (15-oz.) cans red kidney beans
1 tablespoon chili powder
1 teaspoon ground cumin

1 teaspoon dried leaf basil
1 (4-oz.) can diced chilies, if desired,
    drained
2 bay leaves
Hot-pepper sauce
Salt
Freshly ground pepper

In a large saucepan, brown beef without added fat over medium-high heat, stirring to break up meat. Add onion and garlic. Cook, stirring frequently, until onions are softened. Drain off any excess fat. Stir in tomatoes with juice, beans with liquid, chili powder, cumin, basil and chilies, if desired. Add bay leaves. Season with hot-pepper sauce, salt and pepper. Reduce heat, cover and simmer, stirring occasionally, 20 minutes or until onions are tender and mixture has thickened. Discard bay leaves. Makes 6 servings.

Vegetable-Beef Stew

Almost any vegetable can be substituted for those suggested below. Try corn-on-the-cob, cut in 1-inch chunks, winter-squash cubes or rutabaga pieces.

1 tablespoon vegetable oil
1-1/4-pounds lean stew beef, cut in
    1/2-inch cubes
2 large celery stalks, cut in 1/2-inch
    pieces
2 medium-size carrots, cut in 1/2-inch
    pieces
1 medium-size onion, cut in quarters
1 (8-oz.) baking potato, cut in 1-inch
    pieces

2 (4-oz.) turnips, cut in 1-inch pieces
2 cups beef broth
4 cups water
1/4 teaspoon hot-pepper sauce
2 bay leaves
Salt
Freshly ground pepper

In a Dutch oven, heat oil over medium heat. Add beef in batches; sauté until browned. Drain off any excess fat. Add celery, carrots, onion, potato and turnips. Stir in broth, water and hot-pepper sauce. Add bay leaves. Season with salt and pepper. Bring to a boil. Reduce heat, cover and simmer 40 minutes or until meat and vegetables are tender. Discard bay leaves. Makes 6 servings.

Chicken & Vegetables with Peppercorn Mustard Sauce

This recipe can be doubled or tripled easily. It's good with rice or pasta.

2 tablespoons olive oil
8 ounces boneless skinned chicken
  breasts, cut crosswise in 1-inch strips
1 medium-size green bell pepper, cut in
  1-inch strips
1 medium-size carrot, thinly sliced

6 green onions, chopped
1 medium-size tomato, chopped
1/2 cup dry white wine
1 tablespoon green peppercorn mustard
Salt
Freshly ground pepper

In a medium-size skillet, heat olive oil over medium heat. Add chicken. Cook, stirring often, 2 to 3 minutes or until lightly browned. Remove from skillet with a slotted spoon; set aside. Add bell pepper, carrot and green onions. Cook 3 minutes or until vegetables are softened. Reduce heat to low. Return chicken to skillet. Add tomato, wine and mustard. Season with salt and pepper. Cover and simmer until chicken is cooked through and wine is reduced by half, about 5 minutes. Makes 2 servings.

> **Per serving:**
> **259 calories**
> **1.6 grams fiber**

Pineapple Fried Rice

This dramatic presentation will enhance a buffet table. (Photo on page 75.)

1 large pineapple
2 tablespoons vegetable oil
3 green onions, chopped
8 ounces boneless skinned chicken
  breasts, cut in thin strips
1 medium-size green bell pepper, cut in
  thin strips

1 medium-size red bell pepper, cut in
  thin strips
1 teaspoon grated ginger root
Hot-pepper sauce
3 cups cold Basic Brown Rice, page 103
Salt
Freshly ground pepper

Preheat oven to 325F (165C). Cut pineapple in half lengthwise, cutting through green top. Using a small sharp knife, remove fruit. Do not pierce pineapple skin; set pineapple shells aside. Cut 1/2 of pineapple in 1-inch chunks. Reserve remaining pineapple for another use. Wrap pineapple tops in foil to prevent browning. Place on a baking sheet. Bake in preheated oven 10 minutes or until heated through. In a wok or a large skillet, heat oil over high heat. Add onions; stir-fry 1 minute. Add chicken; stir-fry 2 minutes. Add bell peppers and ginger root. Season with hot-pepper sauce. Stir-fry 2 minutes. Add rice and pineapple chunks; stir-fry until hot. Season with salt and pepper. Spoon into hot pineapple shells. Makes 3 to 4 servings.

> **Per serving:**
> **246 calories**
> **2.3 grams fiber**

Chicken & Vegetable Curry

Serve over Basic Brown Rice, page 103, with mango chutney on the side.

1 tablespoon vegetable oil
8 chicken legs, skinned
1 small onion, chopped
1 large garlic clove, minced
2 medium-size carrots, sliced
1 medium-size green bell pepper, cut in
  1/4-inch strips

1 large celery stalk, chopped
2 medium-size tomatoes, chopped
1 cup beer
2 tablespoons curry powder
Salt
Freshly ground pepper
1 (2-inch) cinnamon stick

In a large skillet, heat oil over medium heat. Add chicken; cook until lightly browned. Remove chicken with tongs. Add onion and garlic; cook until onion is softened. Stir in carrots, bell pepper, celery, tomatoes, beer and curry powder. Season with salt and pepper. Add chicken and cinnamon stick. Bring to a boil. Reduce heat, cover and simmer about 25 minutes or until chicken and vegetables are tender. Discard cinnamon stick. Makes 4 servings.

Italian-Style Stuffed Tomatoes

These make a beautiful presentation and have a wonderful flavor.

4 large ripe tomatoes
  8 ounces turkey sausage
  1 large garlic clove, minced
  1-1/2 teaspoons fennel seeds, crushed
  2 tablespoons red-wine vinegar
  1-1/2 teaspoons sugar
  2 tablespoons chopped fresh Italian
parsley

2 tablespoons chopped fresh basil or 2
teaspoons dried leaf basil
1 cup cooked Basic Brown Rice,
  page 103
3 tablespoons pine nuts
2 tablespoons grated Parmesan cheese
Salt
Freshly ground pepper

Cut a thin slice from top of each tomato; remove cores. Using a small serrated spoon, remove pulp; do not pierce sides of tomatoes. Chop pulp; set aside. Drain tomatoes upside down on paper towels. In a medium-size skillet, brown sausage without added fat over medium-high heat, stirring to break up meat. Add garlic. Cook, stirring occasionally, about 5 minutes. Drain off any excess fat. Stir in tomato pulp, fennel, vinegar, sugar, parsley and basil. Cook, stirring occasionally, until mixture is almost dry. Stir in rice, nuts and cheese. Season with salt and pepper. Preheat oven to 375F (190C). Grease a baking dish large enough to hold tomatoes. Stuff tomato shells with rice mixture. Place in greased dish. Bake 20 to 30 minutes or until heated through. Do not overbake or tomatoes will fall apart. Serve hot or at room temperature. Makes 4 servings.

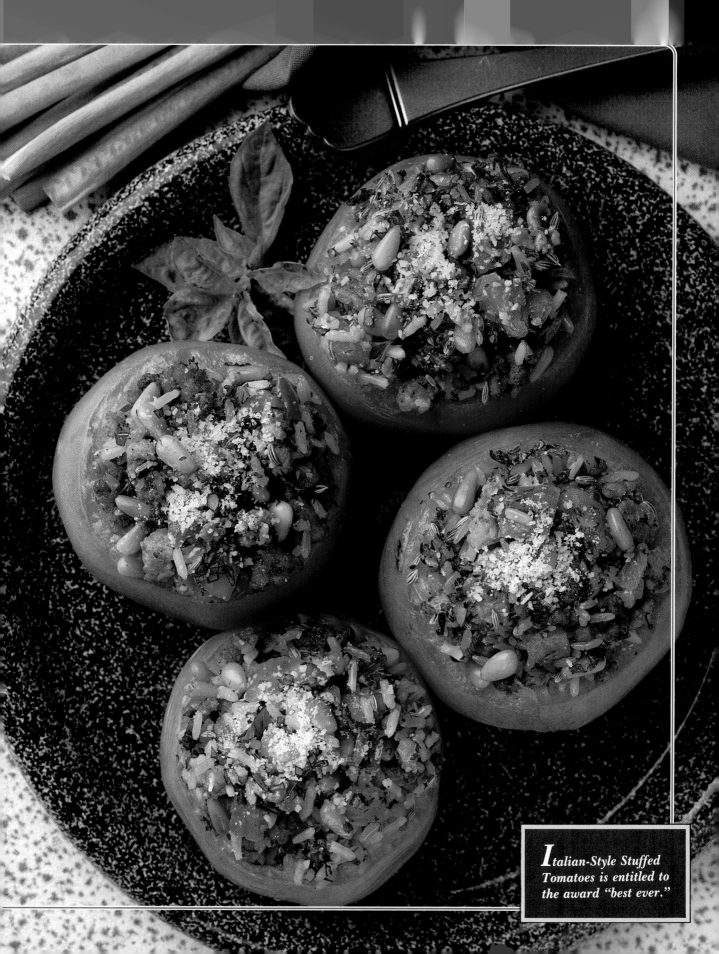

*I*talian-Style Stuffed Tomatoes is entitled to the award "best ever."

Chicken & Pepper Stir-Fry

Stir-frying is quick and easy to do. Have all ingredients near the cooking area before beginning.

6 ounces boneless skinned chicken breasts, cut in 1/4-inch strips
1 teaspoon minced ginger root
1 large garlic clove, minced
1 teaspoon sesame oil
1 teaspoon soy sauce
2 tablespoons vegetable oil
8 green onions, finely sliced

4 ounces Chinese pea pods, cut in 1/4-inch strips
1 large green bell pepper, cut in 1/4-inch strips
1 medium-size zucchini, cut in 1/4-inch strips
6 ounces mushrooms, shredded
Additional soy sauce, if desired

In a small bowl, combine chicken, ginger root, garlic, sesame oil and soy sauce. Heat a wok over high heat. Add vegetable oil and heat until oil is almost smoking. Add chicken mixture; stir-fry until chicken is no longer pink, about 2 minutes. Add onions and pea pods; stir-fry 1 minute. Add bell pepper, zucchini and mushrooms; stir-fry 2 minutes. Season with additional soy sauce, if desired. Makes 2 to 3 servings.

Chicken-Vegetable Bake

Make ahead up to the point of baking. Increase the first cooking time 10 minutes. If red bell peppers are not available, substitute wedges of firm, ripe tomatoes. (Photo on cover.)

6 chicken legs, skinned, if desired
8 ounces pearl onions, parboiled, peeled
8 ounces small mushrooms
1 (15-oz.) can artichoke hearts, drained, cut in halves
1/2 large green bell pepper, cut in 1/2-inch strips
1/2 large red bell pepper, cut in 1/2-inch strips
1 large garlic clove, minced

1 tablespoon chopped fresh parsley
3 tablespoons chopped fresh thyme or 1 tablespoon dried leaf thyme
1/2 cup chicken stock
1/2 cup dry white wine
2 tablespoons all-purpose flour
Salt
Freshly ground pepper
1/2 cup (2 oz.) shredded Monterey Jack cheese, if desired

Preheat oven to 375F (190C). Grease a 2-quart casserole dish. In greased dish, combine chicken, onions, mushrooms, artichoke hearts, bell peppers and garlic. Sprinkle with parsley and thyme; set aside. In a small saucepan, bring stock to a boil. In a small bowl, whisk wine and flour until smooth; stir into boiling stock. Cook, stirring constantly, until thickened. Pour over vegetables (do not pour over chicken). Season with salt and pepper. Cover and bake in preheated oven 20 minutes. Uncover; bake 30 more minutes or until chicken is no longer pink in center. Sprinkle with cheese, if desired. Bake 5 minutes or until cheese melts. Makes 6 servings.

Stuffed Squash

Enjoy forkfuls of cooked squash along with the savory stuffing.

1 (1-1/2- to 2-lb.) acorn squash, cut in
  half lengthwise, seeded
8 ounces ground turkey
1-1/2 cups fresh whole-wheat-bread
  crumbs

1 teaspoon dried leaf thyme
1/2 teaspoon rubbed sage
1 teaspoon salt or to taste
Freshly ground pepper
1/2 cup (2-oz.) shredded Cheddar cheese

Preheat oven to 350F (175C). Lightly grease a 9-inch square baking dish. Place squash cut-side down in greased baking dish. Cover tightly. Bake in preheated oven about 40 minutes or until squash is almost fork-tender. In a medium-size skillet, cook turkey over medium heat until turkey is no longer pink, stirring to break up meat. Drain off any excess fat. Stir in bread crumbs, thyme, sage and salt. Season with pepper. Remove squash from oven; turn cut-side up in pan. Stuff with turkey mixture, mounding stuffing above squash. Bake 20 minutes more or until squash is fork-tender. Sprinkle with cheese. Bake until cheese melts. To serve, cut each squash piece in half. Makes 4 servings.

Per serving:
321 calories
2.0 grams fiber

Chicken-Rice Bake

Serve with a green salad and Oat Bread, page 117.

2 tablespoons olive oil
8 chicken pieces (about 3 pounds)
1 medium-size onion, chopped
2 large garlic cloves, minced
2 cups long-grain brown rice
4-1/2 cups chicken broth
1 teaspoon dried leaf thyme

Salt
Freshly ground pepper
1 (8-oz.) can sliced water chestnuts,
  drained
1 (8-oz.) can artichoke hearts, drained,
  quartered
1 (10-oz.) package frozen green peas

Preheat oven to 350F (175C). In a large skillet, heat olive oil over medium heat. Add chicken; lightly brown on all sides. Remove from skillet. Add onion and garlic to skillet; cook until onion is softened. In a 3-quart flameproof baking dish, combine rice, broth and thyme. Season with salt and pepper. Bring to a boil. Add chicken; cover tightly. Bake in preheated oven 20 minutes. Stir in water chestnuts, artichoke hearts and peas. Cover and bake 20 minutes or until liquid is absorbed and rice is tender. If liquid is absorbed before rice is tender, add additional broth or water as needed. Makes 8 servings.

Per serving:
217 calories
3.6 grams fiber

Oven-Fried Chicken

The yogurt coating keeps the chicken moist and juicy.

1/2 cup plain low-fat yogurt
2 tablespoons Dijon-style mustard
Salt
Freshly ground pepper

4 chicken thighs, skinned
3 tablespoons sesame seeds
2 tablespoons wheat germ
3 tablespoons unprocessed wheat bran

Preheat oven to 400F (205C). Lightly grease a 9-inch-square pan. In a shallow bowl, combine yogurt and mustard. Season with salt and pepper. Coat chicken with yogurt mixture. In another shallow bowl, combine sesame seeds, wheat germ and wheat bran. Dip chicken pieces in wheat-germ mixture; press mixture onto chicken. Place in greased pan. Bake in preheated oven about 40 minutes or until juices run clear when chicken is pierced in thickest part. Serve hot or cold. Makes 4 servings.

Chicken Primavera

High in flavor and fiber!

1 medium-size carrot, cut crosswise in
  1/4-inch slices
1/2 medium-size green bell pepper, cut
  in 1/4-inch strips
4 ounces mushrooms, quartered
1 broccoli stalk, broken in flowerets,
  stem cut crosswise in 1/4-inch slices
2 tablespoons butter or margarine
5 green onions, thinly sliced
1 pound boneless skinned chicken
  breasts, cut in 1/4-inch strips

2 tablespoons all-purpose flour
1-1/2 cups chicken broth
1 cup dry white wine
1-1/2 teaspoons dried leaf basil
Dash hot-pepper sauce
1 medium-size tomato, cut in 8 wedges
2 cups muli-colored rotini (6 oz.),
  cooked, drained
Salt
Freshly ground pepper

In a large saucepan, steam carrot, bell pepper, mushrooms and broccoli over boiling water 5 minutes or until crisp-tender. Remove from pan; set aside. In a medium-size deep skillet, melt butter over medium heat. Add onion; sauté until softened. Add chicken; sauté, stirring constantly, 3 to 4 minutes or until chicken is no longer pink. Using a slotted spoon, remove onion and chicken; set aside. Stir flour into fat remaining in pan; cook about 2 minutes or until bubbly. Stir in broth, wine, basil and hot-pepper sauce. Cook, stirring continuously, until thickened. Stir in tomato, steamed vegetables and chicken mixture. Pour over rotini; toss to combine. Season with salt and pepper. Serve hot. Makes 4 servings.

Turkey & Sauerkraut

Serve with Rye Bread, page 116.

1 (1-lb.) can sauerkraut, drained, rinsed
1/2 small head green cabbage, finely
  shredded
1 small onion, chopped
1 large Granny Smith apple, chopped
1 large garlic clove, minced

2 teaspoons juniper berries, crushed
1 bay leaf
12 small new red potatoes
2 (1-lb.) turkey thighs, skinned
3 cups beer

In a Dutch oven, combine sauerkraut, cabbage, onion, apple, garlic, juniper berries and bay leaf. Place potatoes and turkey over cabbage mixture. Add beer. Bring to a boil over medium heat. Reduce heat, cover and simmer 45 minutes or until turkey and potatoes are tender. Discard bay leaf. Cut turkey in serving pieces. Makes 6 servings.

Per serving:
426 calories
4.3 grams fiber

Chicken-Squash Bake

One three-pound spaghetti squash yields about six lightly packed cups of cooked strands. Extra cooked squash can be refrigerated up to three days or frozen.

1 tablespoon olive oil
1 large garlic clove, minced
12 ounces cooked chicken, cut in 1-inch
  pieces (about 3 cups)
4 ounces mushrooms, sliced
3 cups cooked spaghetti squash
1 (10-oz.) package frozen green peas,
  thawed

3 tablespoons grated Parmesan cheese
1 teaspoon ground leaf thyme
1-1/2 cups tomato sauce
Salt
Freshly ground pepper

Preheat oven to 400F (205C). Grease a shallow 3-quart casserole dish. In a small skillet, heat olive oil over medium heat. Add garlic; cook until garlic starts to brown. In a medium-size bowl, toss garlic, chicken, mushrooms, squash, peas, cheese and thyme until combined. Add tomato sauce. Season with salt and pepper. Toss to combine. Pour mixture into greased dish. Bake, uncovered, in preheated oven about 25 minutes or until hot and bubbly. Serve hot. Makes 4 servings.

Per serving:
330 calories
5.4 grams fiber

Spaghetti Squash with Shrimp Sauce

Spaghetti squash is used instead of regular spaghetti for this delicious combination.

1 (2-lb.) spaghetti squash, cut in half
  lengthwise, seeded
1 tablespoon butter or margarine
1 large garlic clove, minced
1 medium-size red bell pepper, cut in
  1/4-inch strips
1 medium-size zucchini, cut in 1/4-inch
  strips
1 cup dry white wine

1 teaspoon dried leaf basil
Hot-pepper sauce
Salt
Freshly ground pepper
12 ounces cooked peeled shrimp,
  chopped
Chopped fresh parsley
Grated Parmesan cheese, if desired

Steam squash over boiling water about 30 minutes or until squash will separate in strands when probed with a fork. Using a fork, separate in strands; keep warm. In a medium-size skillet, melt butter over medium heat. Add garlic, bell pepper and zucchini; toss to coat with butter. Cook, stirring constantly, about 5 minutes or until vegetables are softened. Add wine and basil. Season with hot-pepper sauce, salt and pepper. Bring to a boil. Add shrimp; heat through. Pour sauce over squash; toss to combine. Sprinkle with parsley. Serve with cheese, if desired. Makes 4 servings.

To cook squash in a microwave oven: Place spaghetti squash halves and 1/4 cup water in a microwave-safe dish. Cover tightly. Microwave on 100% (HIGH) about 7 minutes per pound.

If the fresh fish supply in your area is limited, check the frozen section of your supermarket. Choose packages that are in good condition and show no signs of thawing and refreezing.

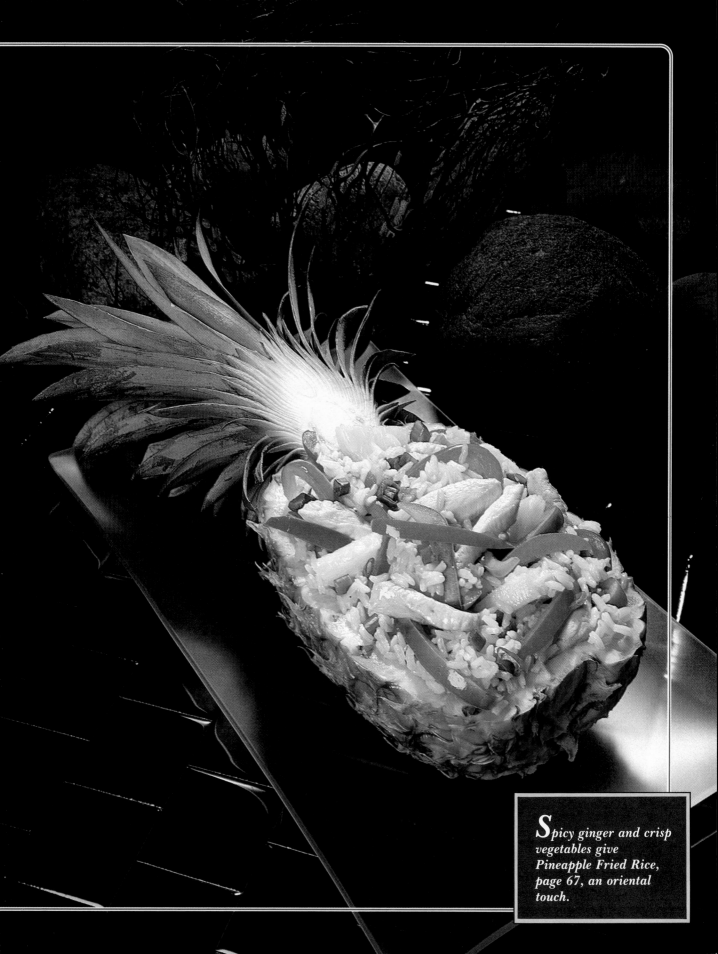

*S*picy ginger and crisp
vegetables give
Pineapple Fried Rice,
page 67, an oriental
touch.

Red Snapper with Tomato Sauce

Serve with Green Beans & Potatoes, page 85, for a quick, nutritious dinner.

2 tablespoons olive oil	1 teaspoon dried leaf oregano
1 medium-size onion, chopped	Hot-pepper sauce
1 small garlic clove, minced	Salt
1/2 medium-size green bell pepper, chopped	Freshly ground pepper
12 ounces tomatoes, chopped	1-1/4 pounds red-snapper fillets (about 1-inch thick)
2-1/2 cups dry white wine	

Preheat oven to 425F (330C). Lightly grease a baking dish large enough to hold fish in a single layer. To make sauce, in a medium-size skillet, heat olive oil over medium heat. Add onion and garlic; sauté, stirring frequently, until onion is softened. Add bell pepper, tomatoes, wine and oregano. Season with hot-pepper sauce, salt and pepper. Bring to a boil. Reduce heat; simmer about 15 minutes or until vegetables are softened but still hold their shapes. Place fish in a single layer in greased dish. Spoon sauce over fish. Bake in preheated oven about 15 minutes or until fish turns from translucent to opaque. Makes 4 servings.

Fish & Vegetables

Cook a fish that doesn't fall apart after cooking, such as monkfish. A large cleaver is ideal for cutting the corn.

2 cups chicken broth	1 pound tomatoes, cut in wedges
2 cups water	1 teaspoon dried leaf basil
8 ounces pearl onions, parbroiled, peeled	1 teaspoon dried leaf oregano
8 ounces zucchini, cut in 2-inch pieces	Hot-pepper sauce
1 medium-size ear of corn, cut in 1-inch pieces	Salt
1/2 medium-size green bell pepper, cut in 1/2-inch pieces	Freshly ground pepper
1/2 medium-size red bell pepper, cut in 1/2-inch pieces	1-1/2 pounds monkfish, grouper, sea bass or other firm white fish, cut in 1-inch pieces
	Chopped fresh parsley

In a large saucepan, bring broth and water to a boil. Add onions, zucchini, corn, bell peppers, tomatoes, basil and oregano. Season with hot-pepper sauce, salt and pepper. Reduce heat, cover and simmer 15 minutes or until vegetables are crisp-tender. Add fish; simmer 5 minutes or until fish turns from translucent to opaque. Ladle into a soup tureen. Sprinkle with parsley. Makes 6 servings.

"Stuffed" Fish

Melted cheese holds the rice together and adds a delicious flavor.

2 tablespoons butter or margarine
1 medium-size onion, chopped
1 garlic clove, minced
2 cups cooked wild rice or long-grain
  brown rice
1 cup (4 oz.) shredded part-skim
  mozzarella cheese
1/4 cup chopped fresh parsley

1 teaspoon salt or to taste
1/2 teaspoon dried leaf thyme
Freshly ground pepper
4 (4-oz.) salmon steaks
Dried dill weed
Parsley sprigs
1 lemon, cut in 4 wedges

Preheat oven to 400F (205C). Grease a shallow baking dish large enough to hold salmon in a single layer. In a medium-size skillet, melt butter over medium heat. Add onion and garlic. Sauté about 5 minutes or until onion is tender; do not brown. Remove from heat. Stir in rice, cheese, chopped parsley, 1 teaspoon of salt and thyme. Season with pepper. Spread rice mixture in greased dish. Place salmon over rice mixture. Season salmon with salt, pepper and dill. Bake in preheated oven about 15 minutes or until fish turns from translucent to opaque. Garnish with parsley sprigs and lemon wedges. Makes 4 servings.

**Per serving:
358 calories
1.1 grams fiber**

Spaghetti with Tuna Sauce

A nice change from the usual tomato-and-meat sauce and quick to prepare.

1 tablespoon olive oil
1 large garlic clove, minced
8 ounces tomatoes, chopped
1/2 cup chicken broth
1/2 cup dry white wine
1 teaspoon dried leaf oregano
1 (6-oz.) can tuna packed in water,
  drained, flaked

1 recipe Whole-Wheat Pasta, page 105,
  cooked
Salt
Freshly ground pepper
2 tablespoons chopped fresh parsley

To make sauce, in a medium-size skillet, heat olive oil over medium heat. Add garlic; sauté until garlic starts to brown. Add tomatoes, broth, wine and oregano. Simmer about 5 minutes or until tomato begins to soften. Stir in tuna; heat through. Place pasta in a serving bowl. Add sauce; toss to combine. Season with salt and pepper. Sprinkle with parsley. Makes 4 servings.

**Per serving:
446 calories
7.3 grams fiber**

Poached Fish with Spinach-Mustard Sauce

This zesty green sauce and mild fish make a perfect combination. Substitute any mild white fish for the orange roughy.

1 thin lemon slice
1 bay leaf

1 pound orange roughy fillets

Spinach-Mustard Sauce:
1-1/2 cups packed fresh spinach leaves
2 tablespoons Dijon-style mustard
Freshly ground pepper

1/2 teaspoon dried leaf tarragon
1 cup plain low-fat yogurt

Prepare sauce; set aside. Fill a large skillet or shallow pan with 2 to 3 inches of water. Add lemon slice and bay leaf. Bring to a boil. Reduce heat to low. Add fish fillets. Cook 3 to 4 minutes or until fillets turn from translucent to opaque. (Cooking time will depend on thickness of fish.) Using a slotted spatula, carefully place fillets on 4 individual plates. Discard bay leaf and lemon slice. Serve with sauce. Makes 4 servings.

Spinach-Mustard Sauce:
In a blender or food processor fitted with the metal blade, process spinach and mustard to a puree. Season with pepper. Add tarragon and yogurt; process only until combined. Makes about 1-1/2 cups.

Tuna Kabobs

Fresh tuna is a very firm fish that barbecues wonderfully.

1 (1-lb.) tuna steak (about-1 inch thick), cut in 1-1/2-inch pieces
16 pearl onions, parboiled, peeled
1 medium-size red bell pepper, cut in 1-1/2-inch pieces
1 medium-size green bell pepper, cut in 1-1/2-inch pieces

1 medium-size chayote, peeled, cut in 1-1/2-inch pieces, parboiled 5 minutes
16 large mushrooms
4 cups hot cooked Basic Brown Rice, page 103

Soy-Ginger Sauce:
1/4 cup low-sodium soy sauce
2 tablespoons seasoned rice vinegar

2 tablespoons honey
1 teaspoon minced ginger root

Prepare barbecue. Prepare sauce; set aside. Alternately thread tuna, onions, bell peppers, chayote and mushrooms on 8 metal skewers.

Brush kabobs with sauce. Grill about 10 minutes or until tuna turns from translucent to opaque. Meanwhile, in a medium saucepan, bring remaining sauce to a boil. Serve kabobs on brown rice. Serve sauce separately. Makes 4 servings.

Soy-Ginger Sauce
In a small saucepan, combine soy sauce, vinegar, honey and ginger root. Stir over low heat until honey dissolves.

Salmon Loaf with Mustard Sauce

For added calcium, do not remove the bones; mash them with a fork and combine with the salmon.

1 (1-lb.) can salmon
1 cup fresh whole-wheat bread crumbs
2 tablespoons unprocessed wheat bran
2 tablespoons lemon juice

1 teaspoon dried leaf tarragon or dried
   leaf dill
Hot-pepper sauce

Mustard Sauce:
2 tablespoons butter or margarine
2 tablespoons all-purpose flour
1 cup low-fat milk
1 tablespoon green peppercorn mustard

1 tablespoon lemon juice
Salt
White pepper

Preheat oven to 350F (175C). Grease an 8" x 4" loaf pan. Pour salmon and liquid into a medium-size bowl; flake with a fork. Stir in bread crumbs, wheat bran, lemon juice and tarragon. Season with hot-pepper sauce. Pack lightly into greased pan. Bake in preheated oven about 35 minutes or until lightly browned. Let stand 10 minutes to firm before slicing. Meanwhile, prepare sauce. Cut loaf in 8 slices. Serve sauce separately. Makes 4 servings.

Per serving:
278 calories
2.0 grams fiber

Mustard Sauce:
In a small saucepan, melt butter over medium heat. Stir in flour. Cook, stirring constantly, until bubbly. Gradually stir in milk. Cook, stirring constantly, until thickened. Blend in mustard and lemon juice. Season with salt and white pepper.

Spinach-Stuffed Fish Fillets

The filling is so delicious that I sometimes double the amount and serve it as a side dish. (Photo on page 60.)

1 tablespoon olive oil	4 ounces spinach, coarsely chopped
1/2 small onion, chopped	Salt
1 small garlic clove, minced	Freshly ground pepper
3 ounces mushrooms, finely chopped (about 1 cup)	4 (5-oz.) red-snapper fillets
1 medium-size tomato, finely chopped	Chopped tomato and green onions, if desired

Per serving:
201 calories
0.9 gram fiber

In a medium-size skillet, heat olive oil over medium heat. Add onion and garlic. Cook, stirring occasionally, about 10 minutes or until onion is transparent. Add mushrooms, tomato and spinach. Season with salt and pepper. Cook, stirring occasionally, until spinach is tender and mixture is dry. Set aside to cool. Prepare barbecue. Spray a fish basket or a piece of foil with nonstick spray. Place fillets on a flat surface. Season with salt and pepper. Divide spinach mixture among fillets, pressing mixture together. Roll fillets, starting at small end. Secure rolled fillets with wooden picks. Place stuffed fillets in basket or on foil. Place on grill; cover with grill lid. Cook about 10 minutes or until fish turns from translucent to opaque. Garnish with tomato and green onion, if desired. Makes 4 servings.

To cook indoors: Preheat oven to 425F (220C). Place stuffed fillets in a lightly greased baking dish. Bake in preheated oven about 10 minutes or until fish turn from translucent to opaque.

Noodles with Eggplant Sauce

This combination sounds unusual but is very good.

2 tablespoons olive oil	1/2 cup dry red wine
1 small onion, chopped	1 teaspoon dried leaf basil
1 large garlic clove, minced	1 teaspoon dried leaf oregano
1/2 medium-size green bell pepper, cubed	Salt
1 (1-lb.) eggplant, peeled, cubed	Freshly ground pepper
1 (28-oz.) can crushed Italian tomatoes	1 recipe Whole-Wheat Pasta, page 105, cooked

Per serving:
488 calories
11.9 grams fiber

In a large saucepan, heat olive oil over medium heat. Add onion and garlic; cook until onion is softened. Stir in bell pepper, eggplant, tomatoes, wine, basil and oregano. Season with salt and pepper. Bring to a boil. Reduce heat, cover and simmer 20 minutes. Serve sauce over noodles. Makes 4 to 6 servings.

Kale & Pork Stew

Serve with corn chips or warm tortillas for a south-of-the-border touch.

2 tablespoons vegetable oil
12 ounces lean pork, cut in 1-inch cubes
1 large onion, coarsely chopped
1 large garlic clove, minced
5 cups water
1 bunch fresh kale, trimmed or 1
  (10-oz.) package thawed frozen kale
1 teaspoon ground cumin

1 dried mild red chili or 1 teaspoon
  chili powder
Hot-pepper sauce
Salt
Freshly ground pepper
1 pound tomatoes, chopped
1 (15-oz.) can yellow hominy, drained

In a large saucepan, heat oil over medium heat. Add pork. Cook, stirring occasionally, 10 minutes or until lightly browned. Add onion and garlic; cook until onion is softened. Add water; bring to a boil. Cut kale crosswise in 1-inch pieces. Add to boiling mixture. Cook, uncovered, until kale is wilted, about 5 minutes. Add cumin and chili. Season with hot-pepper sauce, salt and pepper. Stir in tomatoes and hominy. Cover and simmer 30 minutes or until kale and pork are tender. Discard dried chili, if using. Makes 4 to 6 servings.

> **Per serving:**
> 241 calories
> 4.8 grams fiber

Stuffed Peppers

Serve these hot or at room temperature.

2 tablespoons olive oil
1 small onion, chopped
1 small garlic clove, minced
4 ounces mushrooms, chopped
4 ounces lean ham, finely chopped
  (about 1 cup)
1-1/2 cups cooked Basic Brown Rice,
  page 103

1/4 cup (3/4 oz.) grated Parmesan cheese
2 teaspoons dried leaf basil
Salt
Freshly ground pepper
4 medium-size green bell peppers
1-1/2 cups chicken broth

In a medium-size skillet, heat olive oil over medium heat. Add onion and garlic. Cook, stirring occasionally, until onion is softened. Stir in mushrooms and ham. Cook, stirring occasionally, until mushrooms are tender. Remove from heat. Stir in rice, cheese and basil. Season with salt and pepper; set aside. Preheat oven to 375F (190C). Grease a shallow baking dish large enough to hold peppers. Remove tops, discard core and seeds from peppers. Stuff peppers with ham mixture. Place in greased dish. Pour broth around peppers. Cover with foil. Bake in preheated oven 30 minutes or until peppers are tender. Makes 4 servings.

> **Per serving:**
> 250 calories
> 1.6 grams fiber

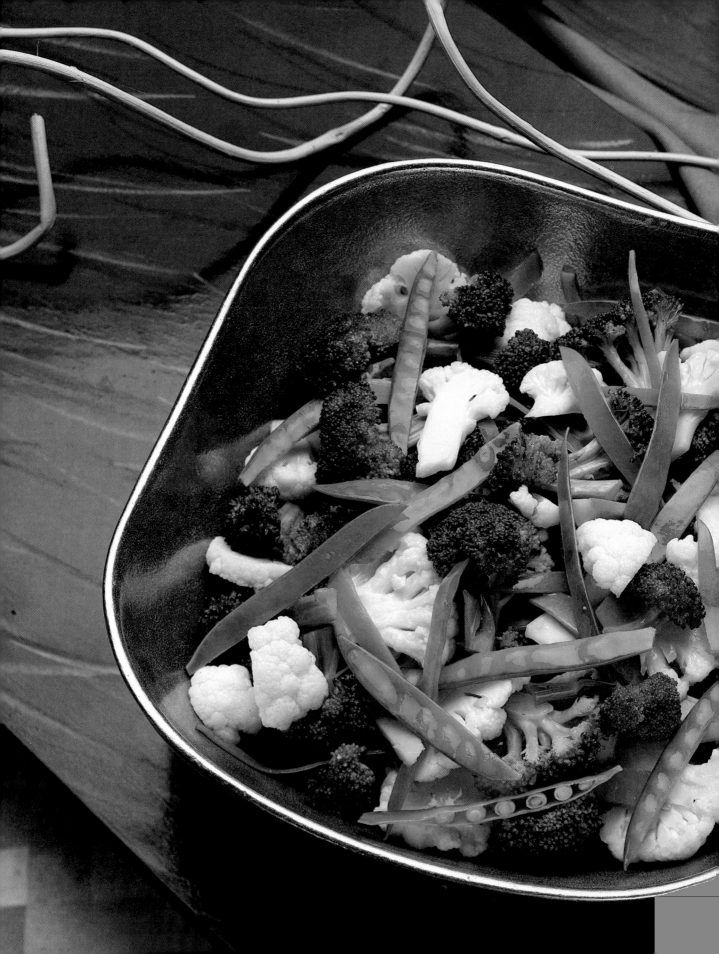

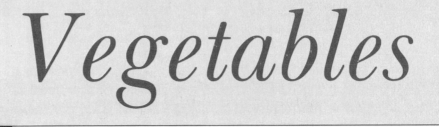

Stir-Fried Vegetables, page 87

Vegetables

CHAPTER FIVE

Vegetables

Did your mother always remind you to eat your vegetables? Well she was right! Not only are vegetables good sources of vitamins and minerals, they also contain fiber, incomplete proteins (proteins missing one or more of the essential amino acids, which are the building blocks for protein) as well as complex carbohydrates. And best of all, except for the starchy vegetables, such as sweet potatoes and squash, vegetables are very low in calories. Even potatoes, which have been falsely accused of being high in calories, are a good source of fiber and vitamin C. The calories come from the butter and sour cream that are usually added.

We have a wider variety of vegetables available to us now than at any time in history. Thanks to rapid transportation many vegetables no longer have a "season" but are available year round. Others disappear for only brief periods. When fresh vegetables are not available, there is an ample supply of frozen and canned vegetables for our selection. Thanks to science and technology, new varieties of vegetables appear each year. Many of these new types are easier to harvest or transport without spoiling.

When buying fresh vegetables, choose firm, crisp, bright-colored vegetables. Avoid vegetables that are limp, have brown spots or signs of decay. If the vegetables you had planned on buying are not at their peak, make another selection—be flexible. Another alternative would be to purchase the vegetable canned or frozen. For example, canned tomatoes can easily replace fresh tomatoes in soups or casseroles.

Use fresh vegetables as soon as possible after purchasing. Refrigerate perishable vegetables. Do not wash vegetables before storing as this causes vegetables to spoil more quickly.

The most important lesson for cooking vegetables is to learn not to overcook them. Most vegetables are at their best when cooked just until tender or until crisp-tender. Quick cooking in steam or a small amount of liquid preserves nutrients, many of which are water soluble. For cooked green vegetables that stay bright in color, bring the liquid to a boil first, then add the vegetables. Let cook without a lid for a few minutes to release volatile acids, then cover for remaining cooking time. Do not add baking soda; it destroys B vitamins and affects the flavor.

Steamed Green Beans

When you buy fresh green beans in the farmer's markets of Germany, a sprig or two of fresh savory, called bohnenkraut or bean weed, is always included without charge.

1-1/2 pounds fresh green beans, ends removed, broken in 2-inch pieces
1 tablespoon chopped fresh savory or 1 teaspoon dried leaf savory

Salt
Freshly ground pepper

In a large saucepan, steam beans and savory over boiling water about 20 minutes or until crisp-tender. Season with salt and pepper. Makes 4 servings.

> Per serving:
> 61 calories
> 3.1 grams fiber

Green Beans & Potatoes

My mother almost always steams the potatoes on top of fresh green beans and reduces the number of pans to wash!

1-1/2 pounds fresh green beans, cut in 1-inch pieces

4 medium-size red potatoes, cut in 1/2-inch slices

Place green beans in a steamer over boiling water. Top with potatoes. Steam about 20 minutes or until potatoes are fork-tender. Season with salt and pepper. Makes 4 to 6 servings.

> Per serving:
> 205 calories
> 3.7 grams fiber

Curried Vegetables

A hint of curry adds an exotic touch. Red potatoes do not break apart as easily as baking potatoes when tossed with the sauce.

2 medium-size red potatoes, cut in 1/2-inch slices
1/2 small head cauliflower, broken in flowerets
1 (10-oz.) package frozen green peas, thawed

1/2 cup chicken broth
1 teaspoon curry powder
Salt
Freshly ground pepper

Layer potatoes, cauliflower and peas in a steamer. Steam over boiling water about 10 minutes or until crisp-tender. Place cooked vegetables in a medium-size skillet. In a small bowl, combine broth and curry powder; pour over vegetables. Cook, stirring gently, over medium heat 2 minutes. Season with salt and pepper. Makes 4 to 6 servings.

> Per serving:
> 148 calories
> 3.9 grams fiber

Lemony Cauliflower & Broccoli

Almost too pretty to eat, but do try this! After it's brought to the table, cut the whole cauliflower in serving pieces.

1 medium-size head cauliflower, trimmed
2 medium-size broccoli stalks, separated in flowerets
1/2 cup chicken broth

2 tablespoons lemon juice
1 teaspoon grated lemon peel
White pepper
Salt, if desired

Cut an "X" in stem end of cauliflower. In a large saucepan, steam cauliflower over boiling water 20 minutes or until crisp-tender. In a medium-size saucepan, steam broccoli over boiling water 8 minutes or until crisp-tender. In a small saucepan, heat broth, lemon juice and lemon peel. Season with white pepper. Taste for seasonings; add salt, if desired. Keep warm. Arrange broccoli around edge of a serving plate with stalks pointing towards center. Place cauliflower in center of broccoli, atop stalks. Drizzle with broth mixture. Makes 6 servings.

Tofu Bake

Tofu, or soybean curd, has a rather delicate flavor. It absorbs the flavors of other ingredients in the dish.

1 (1-lb.) carton tofu, drained, rinsed, drained again, cut in 1/2-inch cubes
1 garlic clove, minced
1 teaspoon low-sodium soy sauce
1 teaspoon sesame oil

1 teaspoon grated ginger root
Freshly ground pepper
1 (10-oz.) package frozen chopped spinach, thawed, well drained
2 medium-size tomatoes, thinly sliced

In a medium-size bowl, gently combine tofu, garlic, soy sauce, sesame oil and ginger root. Season with pepper. Cover; let stand at room temperature 30 minutes. Preheat oven to 350F (175C). Lightly grease a 1-quart casserole dish. Spread 1/2 of spinach in greased dish. Top with 1/2 of tofu mixture. Arrange 1/2 of tomatoes over tofu. Repeat with remaining spinach, tofu and tomatoes. Bake, uncovered, in preheated oven about 30 minutes or until hot and bubbly. Makes 4 servings.

Stir-Fried Vegetables

Don't reserve stir-fried vegetables for Chinese meals. They're equally at home with broiled chicken or fish. (Photo on page 82.)

1 tablespoon vegetable oil
1/2 medium-size head cauliflower, broken in flowerets, cut in 1/4-inch-thick slices
1 medium-size broccoli stalk, broken in flowerets, stem cut crosswise in 1/4-inch-thick slices

4 ounces Chinese pea pods, ends trimmed
Low-sodium soy sauce

In a wok, heat oil over medium-high heat. Add cauliflower, broccoli and pea pods. Stir-fry 2 minutes or until vegetables are crisp-tender. Season with soy sauce. Makes 4 servings.

**Per serving:
133 calories
4.6 grams fiber**

Steamed Vegetable Medley

High in fiber, vitamins and flavor!

1 large broccoli stalk, broken in flowerets, stem cut crosswise in 1/4-inch-thick slices
3 medium-size carrots, cut in diagonal slices

1 (8-oz.) can sliced water chestnuts, drained
1/2 pint cherry tomatoes
2 tablespoons low-sodium soy sauce
1 tablespoon seasoned rice vinegar

In a large saucepan, steam broccoli and carrots over boiling water about 6 minutes or until crisp-tender. Add water chestnuts and tomatoes. Steam about 1 minute or until heated through. Immediately remove from pan; place in a serving bowl. In a small bowl, combine soy sauce and vinegar. Drizzle over vegetables. Gently toss to combine. Makes 4 servings.

**Per serving:
83 calories
3.2 grams fiber**

Sautéed Brussels Sprouts

Quick cooking keeps Brussels sprouts mild-tasting. Overcooking members of the cabbage family gives them a strong flavor.

1 tablespoon butter or margarine
1 pound Brussels sprouts, trimmed, cut lengthwise in thin slices

Salt
Freshly ground pepper
2 tablespoons water

In a medium-size skillet, melt butter over medium heat. Add sprouts; toss to coat. Season with salt and pepper. Add water and cover. Cook, shaking pan occasionally, 4 minutes or until crisp-tender. Makes 4 servings.

Sweet-Sour Cabbage

Vinegar keeps the cabbage's vibrant color. Without vinegar, red cabbage turns blue!

1 large head red cabbage, finely shredded
2 large Granny Smith apples, thinly sliced
1/4 cup water
2 tablespoons red-wine vinegar

2 tablespoons light-brown sugar
1 teaspoon caraway seeds, if desired, crushed
Salt
Freshly ground pepper

In a large saucepan, combine cabbage, apples, water, vinegar, brown sugar and caraway seeds, if desired. Season with salt and pepper. Bring to a boil. Reduce heat, cover and simmer about 10 minutes or until cabbage and apples are tender. Makes 6 servings.

Sweet-Potato Bake

Sweet potatoes have a naturally sweet taste and are high in carotene (a precursor of vitamin A) and fiber.

2 pounds sweet potatoes, peeled, cut in 2-inch pieces
2 tablespoons butter or margarine
2 tablespoons orange-flavored liqueur

1 tablespoon grated orange peel
1/2 teaspoon ground cardamom or cinnamon
2 egg whites

In a medium-size saucepan, cook potatoes in boiling salted water about 20 minutes or until tender. Drain; mash. Beat in butter, liqueur, orange peel and cardamom; set aside. Preheat oven to 400F (205C). Grease a deep

2-quart casserole. In a medium-size bowl, beat egg whites until stiff but not dry. Stir 1/4 of egg whites into potatoes to lighten. Fold in remaining egg whites. Bake in preheated oven about 30 minutes or until puffed and browned. Makes 4 servings.

Sweet-Sour Asparagus

Seasoned rice vinegar is a mild, sweet-tasting vinegar made from rice.

**2 pounds fresh asparagus, ends
   removed, cut in 2-inch pieces**
1 teaspoon cornstarch

1/2 cup chicken broth
2 tablespoons seasoned rice vinegar
1 teaspoon low-sodium soy sauce

In a large saucepan, steam asparagus over boiling water about 15 minutes or until crisp-tender. To make sauce, in a small saucepan, combine cornstarch and 2 tablespoons of broth until smooth. Stir in remaining broth. Bring to a boil, stirring constantly. Cook, stirring constantly, until slightly thickened,. Stir in vinegar and soy sauce. Place asparagus in a serving bowl. Pour sauce over asparagus; toss until combined. Serve hot. Makes 4 servings.

**Per serving:
59 calories
1.8 grams fiber**

Mashed Rutabagas

Serve this high fiber vegetable with roast pork.

**4 medium-size rutabagas, peeled, cut in
   1-inch cubes**
1 tablespoon butter or margarine
About 2 tablespoons low-fat milk

1/4 teaspoon freshly grated nutmeg
Salt
Freshly ground pepper

In a large saucepan, steam rutabagas over boiling water about 45 minutes or until fork-tender. Mash in a medium-size bowl. Beat in butter and enough milk to make a soft consistency. Stir in nutmeg. Season with salt and pepper. Makes 4 servings.

**Per serving:
81 calories
2.2 grams fiber**

Variation
For a milder flavor, substitute 2 medium-size baking potatoes for 1 medium-size rutabaga.

Indonesian-Style Vegetables with Noodles

Hot and spicy, great as a light main course!

2 large carrots, cut diagonally in thin slices

1/2 medium-size head cauliflower, broken in flowerets

2 large green onions, cut in 2-inch pieces

1 large zucchini, cut crosswise in thin slices

1 medium-size green bell pepper, cut in thin strips

1 medium-size red bell pepper, cut in thin strips

Salt

4 cups hot cooked soba or other noodles

Light Peanut Sauce:

1/4 cup dry sherry

3/4 cup chicken broth

2 tablespoons natural smooth unsalted peanut butter

2 teaspoons low-sodium soy sauce

1 garlic clove, crushed

1-1/2 teaspoons grated ginger root

Hot-pepper sauce

3 slices hot red pepper, if desired

Per serving:
325 calories
4.9 grams fiber

Prepare sauce; set aside. In a large saucepan, steam carrots and cauliflower over boiling water 4 minutes. Add green onions, zucchini and bell peppers. Steam 3 minutes or until vegetables are crisp-tender. Season with salt. Arrange vegetables and noodles on 4 plates. Serve with sauce. Sauce can be spooned over each serving or used for dipping. Makes 4 servings.

Light Peanut Sauce:

In a small saucepan, combine sherry, broth, peanut butter, soy sauce, garlic and ginger root. Season with hot-pepper sauce. Cook, stirring constantly, over medium heat until smooth. Garnish with hot pepper, if desired.

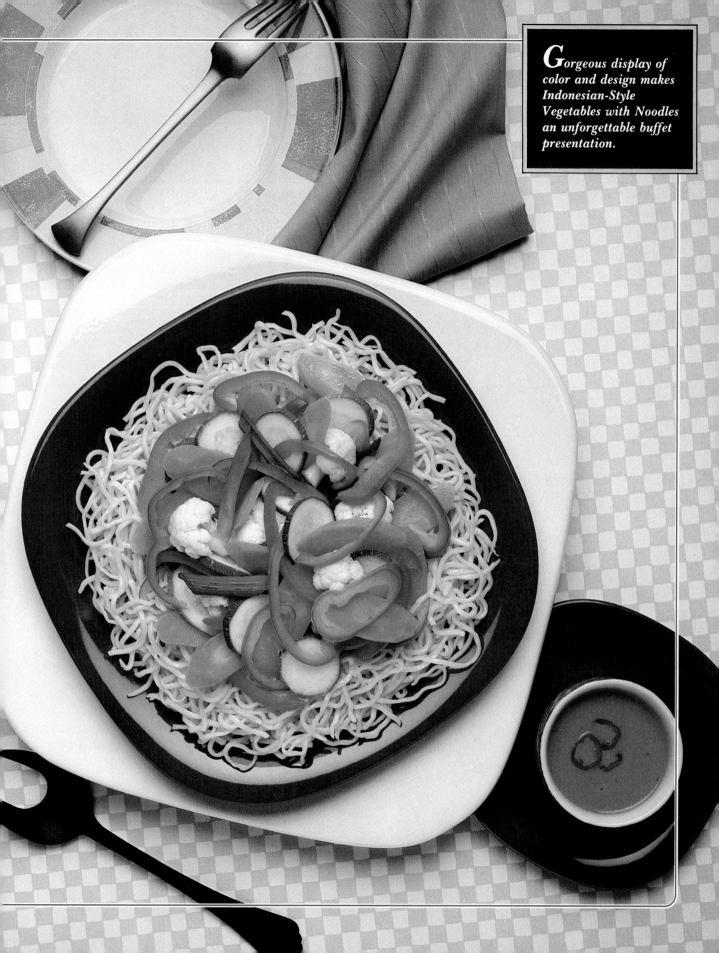

Broiled Tomatoes with Dill-Mustard Sauce

Use vine-ripened tomatoes for the best flavor, but choose tomatoes that are not overripe.

4 large tomatoes
1/2 cup plain low-fat yogurt
1/4 cup mayonnaise
1 tablespoon minced chives

1 teaspoon Dijon-style mustard
1/2 teaspoon dried dill weed
Salt
White pepper

Position oven rack 4 to 6 inches from heat source. Preheat broiler. Cut a thin slice off stem end of each tomato. Place tomatoes, cut-side up, in a baking pan. Broil in preheated broiler about 5 minutes or until hot. Do not overcook. To make topping, in a small bowl, combine yogurt, mayonnaise, chives, mustard and dill. Season with salt and white pepper. Spoon topping over broiled tomatoes. Broil about 1 minute or until warmed. Makes 4 servings.

Herbed Cherry Tomatoes

Quick to prepare, these add bright color to your plate.

1 tablespoon butter or margarine
1 pint cherry tomatoes
1 tablespoon chopped fresh basil or 1
   teaspoon dried leaf basil

1/4 cup chopped green-onion tops or
   chives
Salt
Freshly ground pepper

In a medium-size skillet, melt butter over medium heat. Add tomatoes and stir to coat. Cook, shaking pan gently, 1 to 2 minutes or until tomatoes are hot. Do not overcook. Sprinkle with basil and green-onion tops. Season with salt and pepper. Makes 4 servings.

Orange-Glazed Carrots

Orange sections add a fresh touch.

1 teaspoon butter or margarine
1/4 cup orange juice
3 medium-size carrots, cut diagonally in
   thin slices

1 tablespoon honey mustard
1/4 cup orange marmalade
1 small orange, peeled, sectioned

In a medium-size saucepan, heat butter and orange juice over medium heat. Add carrots. Cover and simmer about 10 minutes or until carrots are crisp-tender. Stir in mustard and marmalade. Cook, stirring constantly, until marmalade melts and mixture thickens slightly. Stir in orange. Makes 4 servings.

Per serving:
167 calories
1.1 grams fiber

Carrots & Chayote

I first had this delicious and attractive combination at the home of my Jamaican friend, Marcelle.

2 large carrots, cut in thin slices
1 large chayote, peeled, cut in 3/4-inch cubes
1 teaspoon chopped fresh mint, basil or parsley

1 tablespoon butter or margarine, if desired, melted
Salt
Freshly ground pepper

In a medium-size saucepan, steam carrots and chayote over boiling water about 15 minutes or until crisp-tender. Place in a serving bowl. Toss with herbs and butter, if desired. Season with salt and pepper. Makes 4 servings.

Per serving:
65 calories
1.8 grams fiber

Zucchini & Carrots

Shredded vegetables have a slightly different texture and cook quicker than whole ones.

1 tablespoon vegetable oil
2 medium-size zucchini, shredded
2 large carrots, shredded

Salt
Freshly ground pepper

In a medium-size skillet, heat oil over medium heat. Add zucchini and carrots. Cook, stirring constantly, about 4 minutes or until vegetables are crisp-tender. Season with salt and pepper. Makes 4 servings.

Per serving:
75 calories
4.1 grams fiber

Variation
Omit salt. To serve, sprinkle with 1 to 2 tablespoons grated Parmesan cheese.

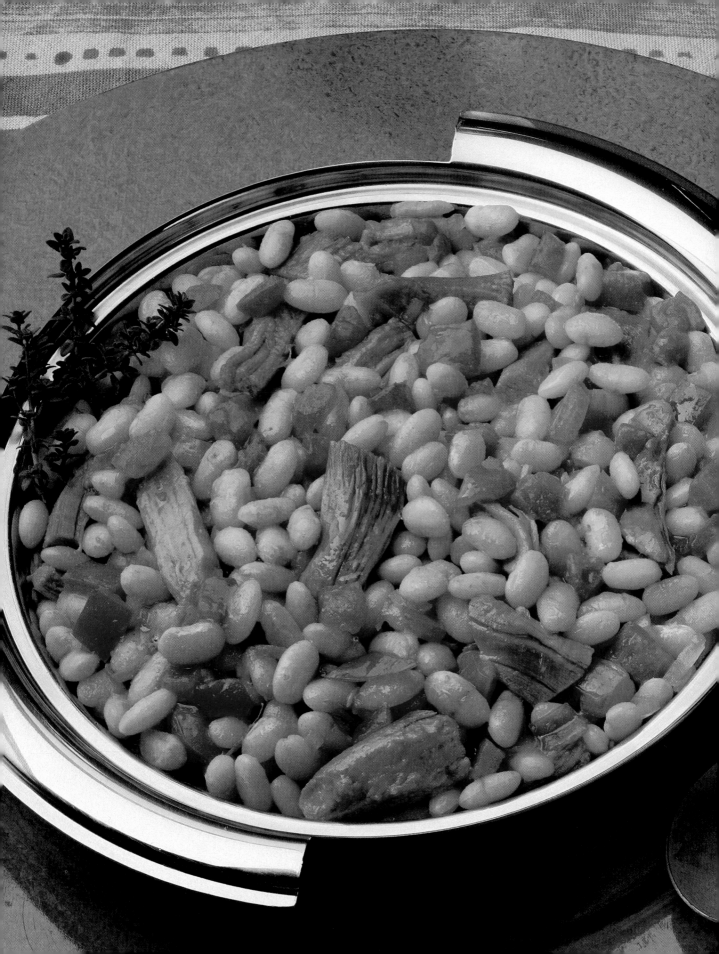

Turkey & Beans, page 99

Beans & Grains

CHAPTER SIX

Beans
& Grains

Beans and grains are the mainstay of the diet for much of the world's population. Many traditional dishes are based on their combination, which results in a supply of complete protein. For example, black beans and rice are a staple in Latin America, beans and tortillas are eaten in Mexico and garbanzo beans and rice are eaten in the Middle East. Early American Indians made succotash, which is beans and corn. For these people, meat is used more as a seasoning than as a main part of the diet. As populations become more Westernized, there is more emphasis on meat and the traditional dishes are considered peasant dishes.

Recently we have learned just how much better for us these peasant foods are! In addition to protein, the beans and grains provide complex carbohydrates, B vitamins and minerals with only a small amount of fat.

If you're short on time, choose some of the canned beans rather than cooking your own. For some beans, such as garbanzo beans and kidney beans, the canned ones are quite acceptable in flavor and texture. Experiment and decide for yourself.

Grains are not so simple to work with as beans. Below is a partial list of some grains, you might want to try.

Barley groats—Unpolished barley kernels.
Brown rice—Unpolished rice that still has part of the outer bran. It is available as long-grain rice and short-grain rice.
Bulgur—Wheat that has been cooked, dried and cracked. It is rehydrated before using in salads or breads. It can be made into a pilaf.
Cracked wheat—Crushed wheat, it is used for cereal and in breads.
Oat groats—Unpolished oat kernels.
Pearl barley—Polished barley kernels.
Wheat berries—Whole kernels of wheat.
Wild rice—Not a true rice, this grass has a nutty flavor. It is the most expensive of the grains.

Garbanzo Beans & Spinach

In the Middle East, cooked dried beans and greens are traditionally combined in soups and main dishes. Serve with hot bread and a salad for a complete meal, or serve as a side dish.

2 teaspoons olive oil	1 (15-oz) can garbanzo beans
1 small onion, chopped	1/2 teaspoon ground cumin
1 small garlic clove, minced	Salt
1 bunch spinach, chopped	Freshly ground pepper

In a medium-size saucepan, heat olive oil over medium heat. Add onion and garlic; cook until onion is softened. Stir in spinach; cook until wilted. Stir in beans with liquid and cumin. Season with salt and pepper. Reduce heat, cover and simmer 10 minutes to blend flavors. Makes 4 servings.

Per serving:
150 calories
5.25 grams fiber

Cuban Black Beans

This dish reminds me of many lunches I enjoyed in Cuban restaurants in Tampa, Florida's Ybor City. Typically served with a green salad and Cuban bread, try it with Whole-Wheat French Bread, page 114, or serve over Basic Brown Rice, page 103.

1 pound dried black beans	1 teaspoon dried leaf oregano
4 cups chicken broth	1 large garlic clove, minced
1 tablespoon olive oil	Salt
1 bay leaf	4 tablespoons chopped onion

Place beans in a large saucepan. Cover with water; soak overnight. Or cover beans with water, bring to a boil and boil 5 minutes. Cover and let stand 1 hour. Drain beans. Rinse saucepan; return beans to saucepan. Stir in broth, olive oil, bay leaf, oregano and garlic. Boil 10 minutes. Reduce heat, cover and simmer about 1-1/2 hours or until beans are tender. Add more water or broth if beans become too dry. Discard bay leaf. Season with salt. Spoon into serving bowls. Sprinkle each serving with 1 tablespoon of onion. Makes 4 servings.

Per serving:
411 calories
4.4 grams fiber

Ranch-Style Beans

Use as a main dish or as a side dish.

1 pound pinto beans
1 tablespoon vegetable oil
1 (4-oz) can diced green chilies
1 small onion, chopped
1 large garlic clove, if desired
1 tablespoon chili powder

1 teaspoon dried leaf oregano
1 bay leaf
6 cups water
Salt
Freshly ground pepper

Place beans in a large saucepan. Cover with water. Soak overnight. Or cover beans with water, bring to a boil and boil 5 minutes. Cover and let stand 1 hour. Drain beans. In a Dutch oven, combine beans, oil, chilies, onion, garlic, chili powder, oregano, bay leaf and 6 cups water. Season with salt and pepper. Bring to a boil; boil 10 minutes. Reduce heat, cover and simmer 1-1/2 hours or until beans are tender, stirring occasionally. Add more water if beans become too dry. Beans should be slightly soupy. Discard bay leaf. Makes 6 servings.

Easy Baked Beans

If using canned beans, taste before adding salt. Serve with Eleanor's Quick Brown Bread, page 120.

2 cups cooked pinto beans, Basic Beans, page 102, or 1 (1-lb.) can pinto beans, drained
2 cups cooked red kidney beans, Basic Beans, page 102, or 1 (15-oz.) can red kidney beans, drained
2 cups cooked navy beans, Basic Beans, page 102, or 1 (15-oz.) can navy beans, drained.

1 (1-lb.) can tomatoes, crushed
1 cup chicken broth
1 small onion, chopped
2 tablespoons dark-brown sugar
2 tablespoons molasses
2 tablespoons cider vinegar
Dash Worcestershire sauce
Hot-pepper sauce
Salt

Preheat oven to 350F (175C). In a 3-quart casserole dish, combine beans, tomatoes with juice, broth, onion, brown sugar, molasses, vinegar and Worcestershire sauce. Season with hot-pepper sauce and salt. Cover and bake in preheated oven 30 minutes. Stir; if mixture is too dry, add more broth or water. Bake, uncovered, 30 minutes more, stirring occasionally and checking amount of liquid. Mixture should be moist but not soupy. Makes 6 servings.

"Refried" Beans

No additional fat is added during cooking. The liquid and stirring prevents the beans from burning. Topped with cheese, these can be the main dish, or serve as a filling for burritos or tacos.

2 cups cooked pinto beans with liquid,
    Basic Beans, page 102, or 1 (1-lb.) can
    pinto beans

Drain beans; reserve 1/2 cup liquid. In a medium-size skillet, heat beans over medium heat. Add reserved liquid. Mash beans until smooth and thick. Continue cooking, stirring constantly, about 5 minutes or until thickened. Makes 2 to 3 servings.

**Per serving:
210 calories
2.9 grams fiber**

Turkey & Beans

A delicious combination that uses the more economical dark turkey meat. (Photo on page 94.)

1 pound dried Great Northern	**1 (1-lb.) skinned turkey thigh**
beans (2-2/3 cups)	**1 medium-size onion, chopped**
1 dried hot red chili	**1 garlic clove, minced**
2 whole cloves	**1 pound tomatoes, chopped**
1 bay leaf	**Salt**
4 cups chicken broth	**Fresh thyme, if desired**
1 tablespoon olive oil	

Place beans in a large saucepan. Cover with water; soak overnight. Or cover beans with water, bring to a boil and boil 5 minutes. Cover and let stand 1 hour. Drain beans. Rinse saucepan; return beans to saucepan. Add chili, cloves, bay leaf and broth. Boil 10 minutes. Reduce heat, cover and simmer 30 minutes. Meanwhile, in a small skillet, heat olive oil over medium heat. Add turkey; brown on all sides. Add turkey to beans. Add onion and garlic to remaining oil in skillet. Cook until onion is softened. Add to beans. Cover and simmer about 45 minutes or until beans are almost tender. Add tomatoes; simmer until beans and turkey are tender. Add more water or broth if beans become too dry. Discard chili, cloves and bay leaf. Remove turkey and cool. Cut turkey in bite-size pieces; stir into beans. Season with salt. Garnish with thyme, if desired. Makes 6 servings.

**Per serving:
333 calories
3.6 grams fiber**

Easy Hoppin' John

There's some debate whether this should be made with red beans or black-eyed peas. However, everyone in the South agrees it should be eaten on New Year's Day for good luck.

4 cups cooked red beans, Basic Beans, page 102, or 2 (15-oz.) cans kidney beans

2 cups cooked Basic Brown Rice, page 103

4 ounces lean ham, finely chopped (about 1 cup)

1 small red onion, chopped

1 tablespoon chopped fresh parsley

1 slice red onion, separated in rings, if desired

Rosemary sprig, if desired

Cilantro sprig, if desired

In a medium-size saucepan, combine beans with liquid, rice and ham. Cook, stirring frequently, over medium heat until hot. Sprinkle with onion and parsley. Garnish with onion, rosemary and cilantro, if desired. Makes 4 servings.

Feijoada

This Brazilian dish sometimes includes salt pork and sausage. These have been omitted to decrease fat. An excellent casserole for a buffet, serve this with a fresh fruit salad.

2 pounds dried black beans

1 pound beef stew meat, cut in 1-inch cubes

1 (28-oz.) can Italian tomatoes

1 large onion, chopped

2 large garlic cloves, minced

8 cups water

Salt

Freshly ground pepper

4 cups cooked Basic Brown Rice, page 103

Place beans in a large saucepan. Cover with water. Bring to a boil; boil 5 minutes. Cover and let stand 1 hour. Drain beans. In a Dutch oven, combine beans, beef, tomatoes, onion, garlic and 8 cups water. Bring to a boil over medium heat; boil 10 minutes, skimming off foam. Reduce heat, cover and simmer 1-1/2 hours or until beans and beef are tender. Season with salt and pepper. Serve with rice. Makes 8 servings.

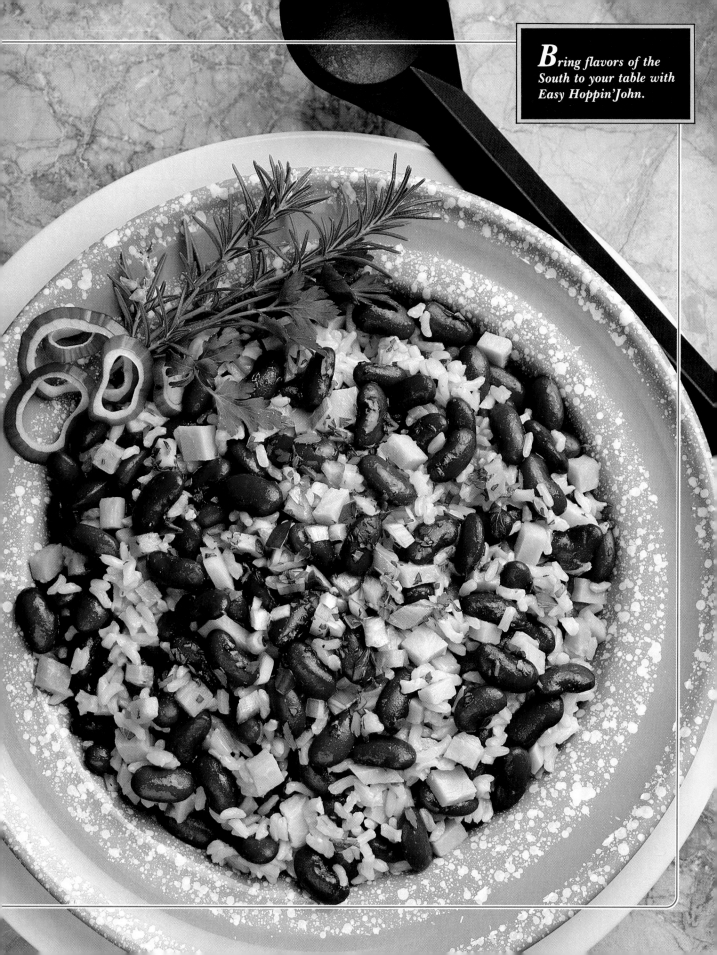

*B*ring flavors of the
South to your table with
Easy Hoppin' John.

Basic Beans

A basic recipe for almost any type of dried bean. Cooking time will vary according to variety of bean and how long it has been stored.

1 pound dried beans
1 tablespoon vegetable oil

1 teaspoon salt
About 6 cups water

Place beans in a large saucepan. Cover with water; soak overnight. Or cover beans with water, bring to a boil and boil 5 minutes. Cover and let stand 1 hour. Drain beans. In a large saucepan, combine beans, oil, salt and 6 cups water. Bring to a boil; boil 10 minutes. Reduce heat, cover and simmer 1-1/2 hours or until beans are tender, stirring occasionally. Add more water if beans become too dry. Makes about 5 cups.

Basic Lentils or Dried Peas

Lentils and dried peas do not have to be soaked before cooking. Use cooked lentils and peas in soups, salads or casseroles.

1 pound dried lentils or dried split-peas
About 7 cups water

1 tablespoons vegetable oil
Salt

In a large saucepan, combine lentils or peas, 7 cups water and oil. Bring to a boil; boil 10 minutes. Reduce heat, cover and simmer until tender. Add more water if mixture becomes too dry. Most liquid should evaporate. Cook lentils about 30 minutes or split-peas about 40 minutes. Season with salt. Makes about 5 cups.

Variation
Substitute 1 pound dried black-eyed peas for lentils. Increase water to 10 cups. Cook about 1-1/4 hours or until peas are tender.

Basic Wild Rice

As a rule, wild rice triples in volume when cooked.

1 cup wild rice
4 cups water

1 teaspoon butter or margarine
1/2 teaspoon salt or to taste

In a medium-size saucepan, combine rice, water, butter and salt. Bring to a boil. Reduce heat to very low, cover and cook about 45 minutes or until rice is tender and water is absorbed. Makes about 3 cups.

Per 1/2 cup:
117 calories
0.7 gram fiber

Variation
Use 1/2 cup wild rice and 1/2 cup long-grain brown rice for a more economical dish.

Basic Brown Rice

Use a nonstick saucepan for easy cleanup. An electric rice cooker will give perfect results. (Photo on page 60.)

2-1/2 cups water
1 cup long-grain brown rice

1/2 teaspoon salt

In a medium-size saucepan, bring water to a boil. Stir in rice and salt. Bring to a boil again. Reduce heat to very low, cover and simmer about 40 minutes or until liquid is absorbed and rice is tender. Makes 4 cups.

Per 1/2 cup:
112 calories
0.7 gram fiber

Variation
Substitute chicken broth for water and omit salt.

Curried Lentils & Bulgur

One cup of dried lentils makes about two cups after cooking. Curry powder adds an exotic flavor.

2-1/2 cups cooked lentils
1/2 cup bulgur
1-1/2 cups chicken broth
2 tablespoons tomato paste

2 teaspoons curry powder
1 teaspoon salt
Freshly ground pepper

Preheat oven to 375F (190C). Grease a 1-quart casserole dish. Combine lentils and bulgur in greased dish. In a small bowl, combine broth, tomato paste, curry powder and salt. Season with pepper. Stir into lentil mixture. Cover and bake in preheated oven about 25 minutes or until liquid is absorbed and bulgur is tender. Makes 4 servings.

Per serving:
241 calories
1.9 grams fiber

Barley-Mushroom Pilaf

Barley is usually reserved for soups. Try this interesting pilaf for a change of pace.

1 tablespoon butter or margarine
1 medium-size onion, chopped
4 cups chicken broth or water
1 cup pearl barley

4 ounces mushrooms, chopped
Salt
White pepper
1 tablespoon chopped fresh parsley

In a medium-size saucepan, melt butter over medium heat. Add onion; cook until softened. Add broth, barley and mushrooms. Season with salt and white pepper. Bring to a boil. Reduce heat to very low, cover and simmer about 40 minutes or until barley is tender and liquid is absorbed. Sprinkle with parsley. Makes 6 servings.

Bulgur Pilaf

A high fiber dish with a nutty flavor.

2 tablespoons butter or margarine
1 small onion, chopped
1 small garlic clove, minced
1 cup bulgur
2 cups chicken broth

1/4 cup chopped fresh parsley
1 teaspoon dried leaf oregano
Salt
Freshly ground pepper

In a medium-size saucepan, melt butter over medium heat. Add onion and garlic; sauté until onion is softened. Mix in bulgur until combined. Stir in broth, parsley and oregano. Season with salt and pepper. Reduce heat, cover and simmer about 25 minutes or until broth is absorbed and bulgur is tender. Makes 4 servings.

Spinach & Brown-Rice Bake

As the cheese melts, it binds all the ingredients together. Serve as a vegetarian main dish or as a side dish.

2 cups cooked Basic Brown Rice, page 103
1 cup cooked spaghetti squash
1 (10-oz) package frozen chopped spinach, thawed, drained

1/2 cup (2 oz.) shredded part-skim mozzarella cheese
Salt
Freshly ground pepper
1/2 cup chicken broth

Preheat oven to 400F (205C). Grease a 2-quart casserole dish. In a large bowl, combine rice, squash, spinach and cheese; toss until combined. Season with salt and pepper. Pour into greased dish; add chicken broth. Bake, uncovered, about 20 minutes or until hot and cheese is melted. Makes 4 to 6 servings.

Per serving: 205 calories 2.9 grams fiber

Variation
Substitute 1-1/2 cups packed shredded summer squash for spaghetti squash.

Whole-Wheat Pasta

Whole-wheat pastry flour, available in natural food stores, can also be used for pasta. Serve with your favorite sauce.

2 cups whole-wheat flour
1 cup bread flour
1/2 teaspoon salt

1 egg
1 tablespoon olive oil
10 to 12 tablespoons water

In a food processor fitted with the metal blade, combine flours, salt, egg, oil and 10 tablespoons of water. Process until dough forms a ball, adding more water through feed tube if needed. Dough should be like a stiff pie dough. Place on a floured surface. Cover and let rest 10 minutes. To make noodles, divide dough in thirds. Roll out 1 piece to about 1/16-inch thickness. Flour well; fold in thirds. Cut in 1/4-inch-wide strips. Unfold noodles; place on a rack to dry. Repeat 2 times with remaining dough. Dry completely or cook fresh. To cook pasta, in a large saucepan, bring 2 quarts salted water to a boil. Add pasta; cook fresh pasta about 1 minute or dry pasta about 10 minutes. Drain. Makes 6 servings.

Per serving: 242 calories 4.5 grams fiber

To make dough without food processor: Pasta can also be mixed and kneaded in a heavy duty mixer. If pasta dough is mixed by hand, knead until smooth. If using a pasta machine, follow manufacturer's directions for rolling and cutting.

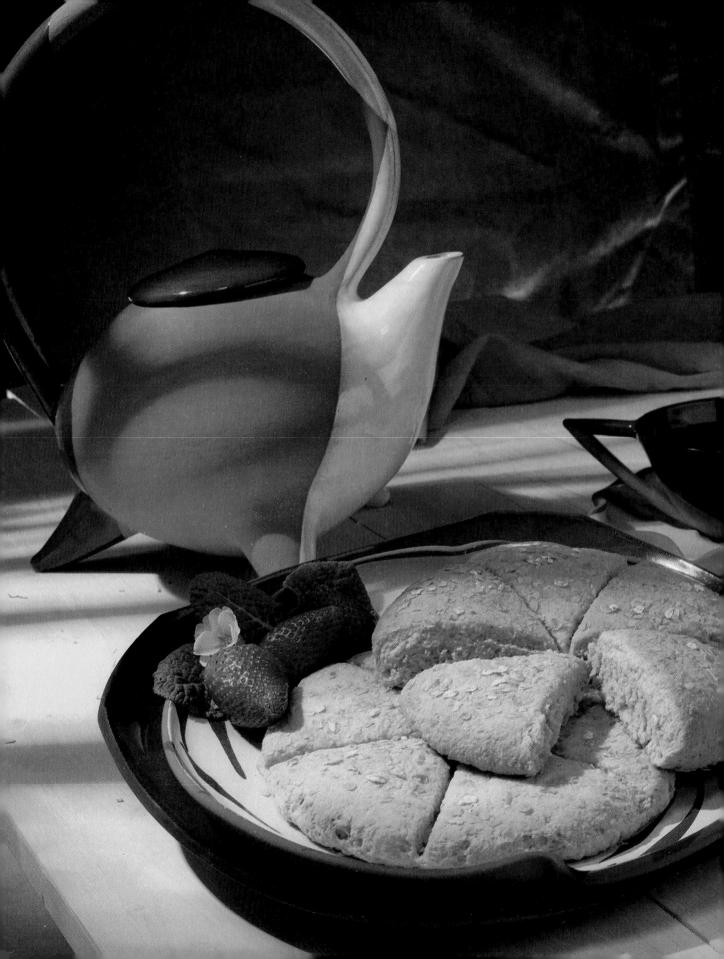

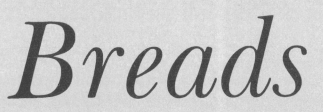

Oat Bran Scones, page 119

Breads

CHAPTER SEVEN

Breads

Nothing gives a warm and homey feeling more than walking into a house and smelling baking bread. Yet many people think that baking bread is too difficult to attempt. They couldn't be more wrong! There are recipes in this chapter for muffins, quick loaf breads, scones, a quick batter bread, standard yeast breads and rolls. By using whole-grain products, such as whole-wheat flour, rye flour, wheat germ and unprocessed wheat bran, it is easy to add fiber to your diet.

Breads can be divided into two categories by the type of leavening agent used to make the bread rise. These categories are quick breads and yeast breads.

Quick breads are leavened by baking powder or baking soda. In addition, air beaten in during preparation and steam from liquid ingredients add additional leavening. Quick breads include muffins, corn bread, scones and pancakes. The method used for most quick breads is the *muffin method*. In this method, all dry ingredients are added to a bowl. All liquid ingredients, such as beaten eggs, vegetable oil or milk are combined and added to the dry ingredients at the same time. The mixture is stirred just until the dry ingredients are moistened. Overmixing results in a heavy product. Biscuits and some other quick breads are made by the *biscuit method*. This is similar to pastry, because the fat is cut into the dry ingredients, then the liquid is added. However, the dough is softer than pastry dough.

As the name implies, yeast is used to leaven yeast breads. Dried yeast is the most commonly available form. When yeast and a small amount of sugar are dissolved in a warm liquid and allowed to stand until foamy, it is called proofing. Adding a small amount of sugar or honey feeds the yeast and makes it grow more rapidly. This gives the yeast a good start before adding it to the other ingredients. It also lets you check if the yeast is active. Discard any yeast that does not start to grow during proofing.

Dissolve dry yeast in liquid that is between 105F to 115F (40C to 45C). Use a thermometer to judge temperature accurately. Too low a temperature will make the yeast grow slowly; high temperatures will kill it.

Yeast dough is kneaded to develop the *gluten*, the protein strands that trap the gas produced by the yeast and gives the baked product its shape.

Kneading can be done by hand or with a heavy-duty mixer with a dough hook. A food processor can also be used to make small amounts of yeast dough, usually about one loaf; do not overprocess.

Let yeast dough rise in a warm, not hot, place that is free from drafts. The ideal temperature is about 80F to 85F (25C to 30C).

Grain Products Used for Baking

All-purpose flour—This is flour from a blend of lower protein wheat. It can be used for yeast breads, quick breads, cakes and cookies.

Bread flour—Flour made from hard wheat. Developed especially for yeast breads, it is high in gluten. Bread flour absorbs more liquid and produces a more elastic dough than all-purpose flour.

Cornmeal—Ground from dried corn, cornmeal is coarser than flour. Available in white, yellow and, recently, blue. It contains both soluble and insoluble fiber.

Oats—Also known as oatmeal or rolled oats, they are high in soluble fiber and low in gluten. Regular rolled oats are higher in fiber than instant rolled oats.

Oat bran—A hot cereal made from oats, it can also be used in baking. It is an excellent source of soluble fiber.

Rye flour—Sifted rye meal, rye flour is available in white, medium (most common) and dark. Dark rye flour has the most fiber. Low in gluten, rye flour should be combined with all-purpose flour or bread flour for baking.

Triticale flour—Made from triticale, which is a grain made by genetically crossing rye and wheat, it is low in gluten. Triticale flour gives bread a nutty flavor. Combine with bread flour or all-purpose flour for baking.

Unprocessed wheat bran—The outer layer of the wheat kernel, it is very high in insoluble fiber.

Wheat berries—The whole kernels of wheat, they can be used as a cereal, sprouted and used in baked products after cooking or sprouting.

Wheat germ—The wheat embryo, wheat germ is high in fat so it must be refrigerated to prevent a rancid flavor. Usually toasted, it adds a nut-like flavor.

Whole-wheat flour—Flour from the whole wheat kernel, it contains both the bran and germ. Used alone, it will produce a heavy, dense bread. It is usually combined with all-purpose flour or bread flour to make a lighter loaf.

Fruit Rolls

Stuffed with fruit, this sweet treat is great for breakfast or brunch.

1 cup low-fat milk
1/4 cup butter or margarine
1/3 cup honey
2 (1/4-oz.) packages active dry yeast
  (5 teaspoons)
1/4 cup warm water (110F/45C)

1 egg, beaten
2 cups whole-wheat flour
About 2-3/4 cups bread flour
2 tablespoons wheat germ
1 teaspoon salt

Filling:
1/3 cup packed light-brown sugar
1 teaspoon ground cinnamon
1/3 cup chopped dried figs

1/3 cup chopped dried apricots
1/3 cup raisins

Per roll:
280 calories
3.6 grams fiber

In a small saucepan, heat milk, butter and honey, stirring constantly, over medium heat until butter melts. Cool to lukewarm. In a small bowl, dissolve yeast in water. Let stand 5 to 10 minutes or until foamy. In a large bowl, combine cooled milk mixture, yeast mixture and egg. Beat in whole-wheat flour, 1 cup of bread flour, wheat germ and salt. Stir in enough remaining bread flour to make a soft dough, about 1-3/4 cups. Turn out dough onto a lightly floured surface. Knead about 10 minutes or until smooth and elastic. Clean and lightly grease bowl. Place dough in greased bowl; turn to coat all sides. Cover with a damp towel. Let rise in a warm place, free from drafts, about 1 hour or until doubled in bulk. Grease a 13" x 9" baking pan. Punch down dough. Cover with a towel. Let rest 10 minutes. Roll out dough to a 16" x 12" rectangle. Prepare Filling; spread over dough to 1-inch from edges. Roll up, jelly-roll style, starting at 1 long edge. Seal edge and ends. Cut in 12 (1-1/2-inch) slices; place in greased pan. Cover with a towel. Let rise about 30 minutes or until doubled in bulk. Preheat oven to 375F (190C). Bake in preheated oven about 20 minutes or until lightly browned. Serve warm or at room temperature. Makes 12 large rolls.

Filling:
In a small bowl, combine brown sugar, cinnamon and fruit.

Applesauce Yeast Braids

This bread is more moist the second day.

2 (1/4-oz.) packages active dry yeast
   (5 teaspoons)
1 teaspoon granulated sugar
1/4 cup warm water (110F/45C)
1 cup unsweetened applesauce
1/2 cup butter or margarine, room
   temperature

2 eggs, beaten
1/4 cup packed light-brown sugar
1 teaspoon salt
2 cups whole-wheat flour
2-1/2 cups bread flour

Cinnamon Mixture:
1/2 cup packed light-brown sugar
1 tablespoon ground cinnamon

1/2 cup chopped walnuts, if desired

Prepare Cinnamon Mixture; set aside. In a large bowl, dissolve yeast and sugar in water. Let stand 5 to 10 minutes or until foamy. Blend in applesauce, butter, eggs, brown sugar and salt. Beat in whole-wheat flour and 1-1/2 cups of bread flour to make a soft dough. Turn out dough onto a lightly floured surface and knead in enough remaining bread flour to make a stiff dough. Clean and lightly grease bowl. Place dough in greased bowl; turn to coat all sides. Cover with a damp towel. Let rise in a warm place, free from drafts, about 1 hour or until doubled in bulk. Grease a baking sheet. Punch down dough. Divide dough in half. Divide each half in 3 pieces. Cover and let rest about 10 minutes. On a lightly floured surface, roll each piece to a 10"x 6" rectangle. Sprinkle each with 1/6 of Cinnamon Mixture. Starting at long edge, roll up, jelly-roll style; seal edges. Place rolls, side-by-side and seam-side down, on greased baking sheet. Braid rolls loosely; seal ends. Repeat with remaining 3 rolls. Cover with a dry towel. Let rise in a warm place, free from drafts, about 30 minutes or until doubled in bulk. Preheat oven to 350F (175C). Bake in preheated oven about 35 minutes or until loaves sound hollow when tapped on bottom. Remove from baking sheet; cool on a wire rack. Wrap in plastic wrap. Let stand at least 8 hours before cutting. Cut each loaf in 12 slices. Makes 2 loaves.

Per slice:
175 calories
1.7 grams fiber

Cinnamon Mixture:

In a small bowl, combine brown sugar, cinnamon and nuts, if desired.

Bran Batter Bread

An easy bread that requires no kneading and rises only once. This can also be beaten with a wooden spoon until smooth and elastic.

1 cup low-fat milk
2 tablespoons butter or margarine
2 tablespoons honey
1 (1/4-oz.) package active dry yeast
  (about 1 tablespoon)
1 teaspoon sugar

1/4 cup warm water (110F/45C)
1-1/2 cups whole-wheat flour
1/4 cup unprocessed wheat bran
1 teaspoon salt
About 1-1/4 cups bread flour

Grease a 2-quart casserole dish. In a small saucepan, heat milk, butter and honey over medium heat, stirring until butter starts to melt. Cool to lukewarm. In a large bowl, dissolve yeast and sugar in water. Let stand 5 to 10 minutes or until foamy. Add milk mixture to yeast mixture. Using a heavy-duty mixer, mix whole-wheat flour, wheat bran and salt into yeast mixture. Beat 2 minutes. Beat in enough bread flour to make a soft dough. Pour dough into greased dish. Cover with a damp towel. Let rise in a warm place, free from drafts, about 45 minutes or until doubled in bulk. Preheat oven to 350F (175C). Bake in preheated oven about 45 minutes or until bread sounds hollow when tapped on bottom. Cut in 10 wedges. Makes 1 loaf.

Sesame-Oat Bread

Sesame seeds add a nutty-flavor and fiber, too! This bread is great for toast.

1 (1/4-oz.) package active dry yeast
  (about 1 tablespoon)
1 tablespoon light-brown sugar
1 cup warm water (11OF/45C)

1 cup regular rolled oats
1/4 cup sesame seeds
1 teaspoon salt
About 2-1/4 cups bread flour

Grease a medium-size bowl. In a small bowl, dissolve yeast and brown sugar in water. Let stand 5 to 10 minutes or until foamy. In a food processor fitted with the metal blade, process oats and sesame seeds until oats are coarsely ground. Add salt and 2-1/4 cups bread flour; process until combined. Add yeast mixture. Process about 5 seconds or until dough forms a ball. Stop machine; check consistency of dough. If dough is too sticky, add additional flour; process until combined. Process dough 15 to 20 seconds to knead. Place dough in greased bowl; turn to coat all sides. Cover with a damp towel. Let rise in a warm place, free from drafts, about 45 minutes or until doubled in bulk. Grease an 8" x 4" loaf pan. Punch down dough. Shape in a loaf; place in greased pan. Cover with a towel. Let rise about 40 minutes or until almost doubled in bulk. Preheat oven to 350F (175C). Bake in preheated oven about 45 minutes or until lightly browned and loaf sounds hollow when tapped on bottom. Remove from pan; cool on a wire rack. Cut in 18 slices. Makes 1 loaf.

To make without food processor: Process oats and sesame seeds in a blender. In a medium-size bowl, dissolve yeast and sugar in water. Make dough as for Whole-Wheat French Bread, page 114.

Wheat-Berry Bread

Wheat berries give a delicious nut-like flavor.

1/2 cup wheat berries
2 (1/4-oz.) packages active dry yeast
  (5 teaspoons)
2 tablespoons honey
2-1/2 cups warm water (110F/45C)

1/2 cup nonfat dry milk powder
1 teaspoon salt
6 cups whole-wheat flour
About 3 cups bread flour

Rinse a thermos with boiling water. Add wheat berries and 2 cups boiling water to thermos. Seal and let stand overnight. Or in a medium-size saucepan, combine wheat berries and 2 cups water. Cover and cook over low heat 2 hours or until tender. Add more water as needed. Drain wheat berries; set aside. In a large bowl, dissolve yeast and honey in 1/2 cup of water. Let stand 5 to 10 minutes or until foamy. Stir in wheat berries, remaining 2 cups of water, milk, salt and 2 cups of whole-wheat flour. Stir in remaining whole-wheat flour and enough bread flour to make a moderately stiff dough. Turn out dough onto a floured surface. Knead about 10 minutes or until smooth and satiny. Clean and lightly grease bowl. Place dough in greased bowl; turn to coat all sides. Cover with a damp towel. Let rise in a warm place, free from drafts, about 1 hour or until doubled in bulk. Grease 2 (9" x 5") loaf pans. Punch down dough. Shape in 2 loaves; place in greased pans. Cover with a towel. Let rise about 40 minutes or until doubled in bulk. Preheat oven to 350F (175C). Bake in preheated oven about 40 minutes or until loaves are browned and sound hollow when tapped on bottom. Remove from pans; cool on wire racks. Cut each loaf in 18 slices. Makes 2 large loaves.

Per slice:
110 calories
2.3 grams fiber

Wild-Rice Bread

Wild rice gives this bread a nutty, exotic taste.

2 (1/4-oz.) packages active dry yeast
  (5 teaspoons)
2 tablespoons honey
2-1/2 cups warm water (110F/45C)
1-1/2 cups cooked Basic Wild Rice,
  page 103

1 teaspoon salt
5 cups whole-wheat flour
About 3 cups bread flour

Per slice:
100 calories
2.0 grams fiber

In a large bowl, dissolve yeast and honey in 1/2 cup of water. Let stand 5 to 10 minutes or until foamy. Stir in remaining 2 cups of water, rice, salt and 2 cups of whole-wheat flour. Stir in remaining whole-wheat flour and enough bread flour to make a moderately stiff dough. Turn out dough onto a floured surface. Knead about 10 minutes or until smooth and satiny. Clean and lightly grease bowl. Place dough in greased bowl; turn to coat all sides. Cover with a damp towel. Let rise in a warm place, free from drafts, about 1 hour or until doubled in bulk. Grease 2 (9" x 5") loaf pans. Punch down dough. Shape in 2 loaves; place in greased pans. Cover with a towel. Let rise about 40 minutes or until doubled in bulk. Preheat oven to 350F (175C). Bake in preheated oven about 40 minutes or until loaves are browned and sound hollow when tapped on bottom. Remove from pans; cool on wire racks. Cut each loaf in 18 slices. Makes 2 loaves.

Whole-Wheat French Bread

If you do not have French bread pans, bake the loaves on large baking sheets. If using shiny bread pans, turn baked loaves over and bake an additional 5 minutes to brown bottoms. (Photo on cover.)

3-1/2 teaspoons active dry yeast
1-1/2 teaspoons light-brown sugar
1-1/2 cups warm water (110F/45C)
2 tablespoons butter or margarine, room
  temperature

1-1/4 teaspoons salt
2 tablespoons unprocessed wheat bran
2 tablespoons wheat germ
2-2/3 cups whole-wheat flour
About 1-1/4 cups bread flour

Per slice:
70 calories
1.5 grams fiber

In a medium-size bowl, dissolve yeast and brown sugar in water. Let stand 5 to 10 minutes or until foamy. Stir butter, salt, wheat bran and wheat germ into yeast mixture. Stir in whole-wheat flour. Stir in enough bread flour to make a moderately stiff dough. Turn out dough onto a floured surface. Knead about 10 minutes or until smooth and elastic. Clean and lightly grease bowl. Place dough in greased bowl; turn to coat all sides.

Cover with a damp towel. Let rise in a warm place, free from drafts, about 45 minutes or until doubled in bulk. Grease 2 French bread pans. Punch down dough. Shape in 2 (12-inch) long loaves; place in greased pans. Cover with a towel. Let rise about 35 minutes or until doubled in bulk. Diagonally cut 2 or 3 slashes, about 1/4 inch deep, in top of loaf. Preheat oven to 400F (205C). Bake in preheated oven about 20 minutes or until bread is crispy and sounds hollow when tapped on bottom. Cut each loaf in 14 slices. Makes 2 loaves.

Variation
Brush loaves with water before baking. Sprinkle with sesame seeds, caraway seeds or poppy seeds, lightly pressing seeds into dough.

Middle Eastern Flat Bread

This bread does not puff like pita bread, but it is light and about 1/2-inch thick. It can be sliced in half and used for sandwiches or as a quick pizza crust.

1 (1/4-oz.) package active dry yeast
   (about 1 tablespoon)
2 teaspoons light-brown sugar
1-1/2 cups warm water (110F, 45C)

3 cups whole-wheat flour
1/2 teaspoon salt
About 1 cup bread flour
Cornmeal

Per round:
150 calories
4.0 grams fiber

In a medium-size bowl, dissolve yeast and brown sugar in water. Let stand 5 to 10 minutes or until foamy. Beat in whole-wheat flour and salt. Stir in enough bread flour to make a moderately stiff dough. Use remaining flour on board. Turn out dough onto a floured surface. Knead about 10 minutes or until smooth and elastic. Clean and lightly grease bowl. Place dough in bowl; turn to coat all sides. Cover with a damp towel. Let rise in a warm place, free from drafts, about 45 minutes or until doubled in bulk. Punch down dough. Shape in 8 balls. On a lightly floured surface, roll out each ball to a 6-inch circle about 1/4-inch thick. Cover with a towel. Let rise about 20 minutes or until almost doubled in bulk. Position oven racks in 2 center positions. Preheat oven to 425F (220C). Grease 2 baking sheets. Place 2 dough rounds on each greased baking sheet. Set 1 baking sheet on lower oven rack. Bake in preheated oven 5 minutes. Move baking sheet to upper rack; place remaining baking sheet on lower rack. Bake 5 more minutes or until bread on upper rack is lightly browned on bottom. Remove baking sheet from upper rack. Move baking sheet on lower rack to upper rack. Repeat with remaining 4 dough rounds. As bread is removed from oven, wrap in foil. Let stand about 15 minutes to soften. Remove from foil; cool completely. Makes 8 (6-inch) round loaves.

Rye Bread

The beer, caraway seeds and orange peel give this bread a delightful flavor. Rye flour tends to makes this dough sticky and slightly harder to work with.

1 (1/4-oz.) package active dry yeast
  (about 1 tablespoon)
1 tablespoon light-brown sugar
1/4 cup warm water (110F/45C)
2 cups rye flour
2 cups bread flour
2 tablespoons unprocessed wheat bran

1/2 teaspoon salt
2 tablespoons caraway seeds, crushed
1 tablespoon grated orange peel
1 cup beer, room temperature
2 tablespoons molasses
2 tablespoons vegetable shortening

Grease a medium-size bowl. In a small bowl, dissolve yeast and brown sugar in water. Let stand 5 to 10 minutes or until foamy. In a food processor fitted with the metal blade, combine flours, wheat bran, salt, caraway seeds and orange peel. Add yeast mixture, beer and molasses. Process until dough forms a ball. Stop machine; check dough for consistency. If too sticky, add additional flour; process until combined. Process dough 15 to 20 seconds to knead. Place dough in greased bowl; turn to coat all sides. Cover with a damp towel. Let rise in a warm place, free from drafts, 45 minutes or until doubled in bulk. Grease a baking sheet. Punch down dough. Shape dough in a 6-inch round loaf. Place on greased baking sheet. Cover with a towel. Let rise about 30 minutes or until almost doubled in bulk. Using a sharp knife or a razor blade, slash top of loaf 3 times. Preheat oven to 375F (190C). Bake in preheated oven about 50 minutes or until loaf sounds hollow when tapped on bottom. Cool on a wire rack. Cut in 16 slices. Makes 1 loaf.

To make without food processor: In a medium-size bowl, dissolve yeast and sugar in warm water. Make dough as for Whole-Wheat French Bread, page 114.

Oat Bread

This bread combines the flavor of oats and wheat into a wonderful bread for sandwiches.

1 cup regular rolled oats
2 cups low-fat milk, scalded
1/3 cup packed light-brown sugar
2 teaspoons salt
1 (1/4-oz.) package active dry yeast
  (about 1 tablespoon)
1 teaspoon brown sugar

1/4 cup warm water (110F/45C)
1/4 cup vegetable oil
1 egg, beaten
3 cups triticale flour or whole-wheat
  flour
3 to 4 cups bread flour

In a large bowl, combine oats, milk, 1/3 cup brown sugar and salt. Let stand until lukewarm. In a small bowl, dissolve yeast and 1 teaspoon brown sugar in water. Let stand 5 to 10 minutes or until foamy. Stir yeast mixture, oil and egg into oat mixture. Beat in triticale flour. Stir in enough bread flour to make a moderately stiff dough. Turn out dough onto a floured surface. Knead about 10 minutes or until smooth and elastic. Clean and lightly grease bowl. Place dough in greased bowl; turn to coat all sides. Cover with a damp towel. Let rise in a warm place, free from drafts, about 1 hour or until doubled in bulk. Grease 2 (9" x 5") loaf pans. Punch down dough. Shape in 2 loaves; place in greased pans. Cover with a towel. Let rise about 1 hour or until doubled in bulk. Preheat oven to 350F (175C). Bake in preheated oven about 50 minutes or until loaves sounds hollow when tapped on bottom. Cool on a wire rack. Cut each loaf in 18 slices. Makes 2 large loaves.

Per slice:
117 calories
2.6 grams fiber

Whole-Wheat Potato Rolls

Potatoes keep these rolls soft and moist.

2 medium-size baking potatoes, peeled,
 chopped
2 cups water
2 (1/4-oz.) packages active dry yeast (5
 teaspoons)
1/4 cup butter or margarine

3 tablespoons honey
2 eggs, lightly beaten
About 4 cups bread flour
4 cups whole-wheat flour
2 teaspoons salt

**Per roll:
110 calories
2.7 grams fiber**

In a medium-size saucepan, boil potatoes in water about 20 minutes or until fork-tender. Drain potatoes, reserving water. Transfer potatoes to a large bowl and mash. Stir in butter and honey. Cool to lukewarm. In a small bowl, dissolve yeast in 1/2 cup of warm potato water. Let stand 5 to 10 minutes or until foamy. Add yeast mixture and eggs to potato mixture; beat until combined. Add enough water to remaining potato water to make 1-1/2 cups; stir into potato mixture. Beat in 2 cups of bread flour. Beat in whole-wheat flour. Stir in enough remaining bread flour to make a soft dough. Turn out dough onto a lightly floured surface. Knead about 10 minutes or until smooth and satiny. Clean and lightly grease bowl. Place dough in greased bowl; turn to coat all sides. Cover with a damp towel. Let rise in a warm place, free from drafts, about 1 hour or until doubled in bulk. Grease 24 (2-1/2- to 3-inch) muffin cups. Punch down dough. Shape dough in 24 balls; place in greased muffin cups. Cover with a towel. Let rise about 30 minutes or until doubled in bulk. Preheat oven to 425F (220C). Bake rolls in preheated oven about 12 minutes or until lightly browned. Makes 24 rolls.

Oat Bran Scones

Serve hot for tea or lunch.

1 cup all-purpose flour
1 tablespoon baking powder
1/4 teaspoon salt
1 cup oat bran
2 tablespoons light-brown sugar

1/4 cup butter or margarine, chilled, chopped
About 2/3 cup low-fat milk
1/4 cup regular rolled oats

Preheat oven to 425F (220C). Grease a baking sheet. Sift flour, baking powder and salt into a medium-size bowl. Stir in oat bran and brown sugar. Using 2 knives or a pastry blender, cut in butter until mixture resembles coarse crumbs. Stir in enough milk to make a soft dough. Turn out dough onto a lightly floured surface. Knead until smooth. Divide dough in half. Sprinkle 1/2 of oats on floured surface. Roll out 1 piece of dough to a 5-1/2-inch circle 3/4-inch thick. Pat some oats on dough. Place on greased baking sheet. Repeat with remaining dough. Mark each circle in 6 equal wedges, cutting almost through. Bake in preheated oven about 18 minutes or until browned. Break wedges apart. Makes 12 scones.

Per scone:
100 calories
1.3 grams fiber

Sweet-Potato Biscuits

These biscuits don't need jam; they're already sweet. If you want them less sweet, reduce the brown sugar to 1 tablespoon.

1-1/4 cups all-purpose flour
1 tablespoon baking powder
1/4 teaspoon salt
1 cup oat bran

2 tablespoons light-brown sugar
1/4 cup butter or margarine, chilled
1/2 cup mashed cooked sweet potatoes
1/4 cup low-fat milk

Preheat oven to 425F (220C). Grease a baking sheet. Sift flour, baking powder and salt into a medium-size bowl. Stir in oat bran and brown sugar. Using 2 knives or a pastry blender, cut in butter until mixture resembles coarse crumbs. Stir in sweet potatoes and milk to make a soft dough. Turn out dough onto a lightly floured board. Knead lightly until smooth. Roll out dough 1/2-inch thick. Cut 14 rounds with a 2-1/4-inch round cutter. Place on greased baking sheet. Bake in preheated oven about 18 minutes or until lightly browned. Makes 14 biscuits.

Per biscuit:
110 calories
1.3 grams fiber

Banana Bread

A heavy, moist bread with a distinct banana flavor.

1 cup unbleached all-purpose flour
2 teaspoons baking powder
1/2 teaspoon ground cinnamon
1/4 teaspoon ground cloves
1/4 teaspoon salt
3/4 cup oat bran

2 eggs
2/3 cup packed light-brown sugar
1/3 cup vegetable oil
3 medium-size ripe bananas, mashed
   (about 1-1/2 cups)

Preheat oven to 350F (175C). Grease a 9" x 5" loaf pan. Sift flour, baking powder, cinnamon, cloves and salt into a medium-size bowl. Stir in oat bran; set aside. In another medium-size bowl, lightly beat eggs. Add brown sugar and oil; beat until combined. Beat in bananas. Add dry ingredients to banana mixture; beat just until combined. Pour into greased pan. Bake in preheated oven about 50 minutes or until bread is browned and top springs back when lightly pressed. Remove from pan; cool on a wire rack. Cut in 18 slices. Makes 1 loaf.

Eleanor's Quick Brown Bread

Don't be alarmed by the thin batter. This rich, sweet bread was first introduced to me by my friend Eleanor. This is a bread I'm sure you'll like.

1/4 cup packed dark-brown sugar
1/4 cup molasses
3 tablespoons vegetable oil
2 cups low-fat milk
2 cups whole-wheat flour

1/2 cup oat bran
1/2 cup all-purpose flour
1 teaspoon baking soda
1/4 teaspoon salt

Preheat oven to 350F (175C). Grease 2 (14" x 8") loaf pans. In a medium-size bowl, combine brown sugar, molasses, oil and milk. In another medium-size bowl, combine whole-wheat flour and oat bran. Sift in all-purpose flour, baking soda and salt. Stir to combine. Stir flour mixture into milk mixture just until combined. Pour batter into greased pans. Cover tightly with foil. Bake in preheated oven about 45 minutes or until top springs back when lightly pressed. Remove from pans. Cool slightly on wire racks. Cut in 16 slices. Serve warm. Makes 2 loaves.

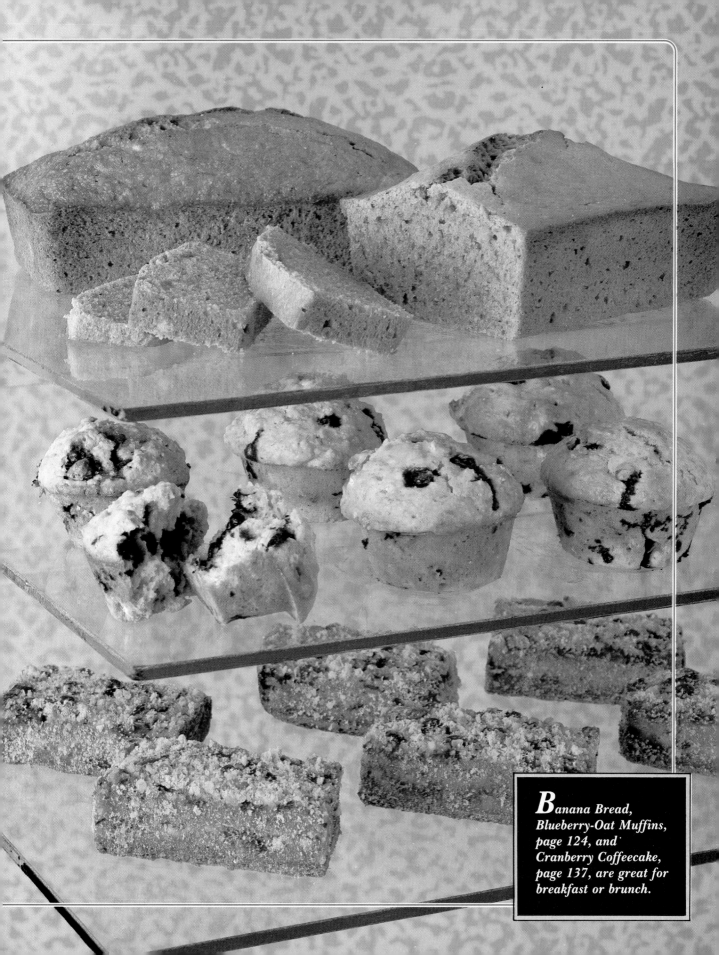

*B*anana Bread, Blueberry-Oat Muffins, page 124, and Cranberry Coffeecake, page 137, are great for breakfast or brunch.

Blue-Corn Bread

The combination of grains add a delightful texture to this bread. Blue cornmeal is available in speciality stores or by mail order. Substitute regular or stone-ground yellow cornmeal, if desired.

1-1/2 cups blue cornmeal
3/4 cup whole-wheat flour
2 tablespoons unprocessed wheat bran
2 tablespoons wheat germ
2 teaspoons baking powder

1/2 teaspoon baking soda
1/2 teaspoon salt
1 egg
2 tablespoons vegetable oil
2 cups buttermilk

Preheat oven to 425F (220C). Grease a 9-inch-square pan. In a medium-size bowl, combine cornmeal, flour, wheat bran and wheat germ. Sift in baking powder, baking soda and salt; stir to combine. In another medium-size bowl, beat egg. Add oil and buttermilk. Beat until combined. Add liquid ingredients to dry ingredients. Stir until dry ingredients are just moistened. Pour into greased pan. Bake in preheated oven about 30 minutes or until a wooden pick inserted in center comes out clean. Cut in 8 pieces. Makes 8 servings.

Double-Corn Bread

Serve with cooked dried beans and cole slaw for a complete meal.

1 cup all-purpose flour
1 tablespoon baking powder
1/2 teaspoon salt
1 cup cornmeal
1 egg
1 (12-oz.) can whole-kernel corn,
   drained

2 tablespoon vegetable oil
1-1/4 cups low-fat milk
1/4 cup diced canned chilies, if desired,
   drained

Preheat oven to 400F (205C). Grease a 9-inch-square baking pan. Sift flour, baking powder and salt into a medium-size bowl. Stir in cornmeal. In another medium-size bowl, lightly beat egg. Stir in corn, oil, milk and chilies, if desired. Stir milk mixture into dry ingredients just until dry ingredients are moistened; mixture will be lumpy. Pour into greased pan. Bake in preheated oven about 40 minutes or until top springs back when lightly pressed. Cut in 8 pieces. Makes 8 servings.

Grated Corncakes

When I was growing up, these were one of my favorite summer foods. This is my version of my mother's recipe.

3/4 cup all-purpose flour
2 teaspoons baking powder
1/2 teaspoon salt
2 eggs

1-1/2 cups grated fresh corn (about 3 small ears)
1/2 cup low-fat milk
2 tablespoons vegetable oil

Preheat a griddle over medium heat. Sift flour, baking powder and salt into a medium-size bowl. In another medium-size bowl, beat eggs. Add corn, milk and oil. Beat until combined. Stir in dry ingredients until combined. Lightly grease hot griddle or coat with vegetable spray. Drop batter by 1/4-cupfuls onto preheated griddle. Cook until edges are bubbly. Turn; cook until lightly browned and centers are cooked through, about 5 minutes total cooking time. Makes 10 corncakes.

Per corncake:
115 calories
1.0 gram fiber

Whole-Wheat Squash Bread

Use leftover spaghetti squash for this spicy quick bread.

1 egg
1 cup low-fat milk
2 tablespoons vegetable oil
1/2 cup packed light-brown sugar
1 cup all-purpose flour
1 teaspoon ground cinnamon

1/2 teaspoon ground allspice
1 tablespoon baking powder
1/2 teaspoon salt
1 cup whole-wheat flour
1 cup packed spaghetti squash
1 cup raisins

Preheat oven to 350F (175C). Grease a 9" x 5" loaf pan. In a medium-size bowl, beat egg. Beat in milk, oil and brown sugar. Sift all-purpose flour, cinnamon, allspice, baking powder and salt into another medium-size bowl. Stir in whole-wheat flour. Stir milk mixture into dry ingredients; beat just until combined. Stir in squash and raisins. Pour into greased pan. Bake in preheated oven about 50 minutes or until a wooden pick inserted in center comes out clean. Let cool in pan on a wire rack 10 minutes. Turn out on a wire rack to cool completely. Cut in 18 slices. Makes 1 loaf.

Per slice:
123 calories
1.2 grams fiber

Blueberry-Oat Muffins

Chopped dried fruit or raisins can be substituted for the blueberries. (Photo on page 121.)

1-1/4 cups all-purpose flour
2-1/2 teaspoons baking powder
1/4 teaspoon salt
3/4 cup regular rolled oats
1 tablespoon unprocessed wheat bran
1/4 cup plus 1 tablespoon packed
   light-brown sugar

1 egg
1/4 cup vegetable oil
1-1/4 cups low-fat milk
3/4 cup fresh or thawed frozen
   blueberries

Per muffin:
160 calories
1.5 grams fiber

Preheat oven to 400F (205C). Grease 12 (2-1/2-to 3-inch) muffin cups. Sift flour, baking powder and salt into a medium-size bowl. Stir in oats, wheat bran and brown sugar; set aside. In a small bowl, beat egg. Mix in oil and milk. Stir milk mixture into dry ingredients just until moistened. Gently stir in blueberries. Spoon batter into greased muffin cups, filling each 2/3 full. Bake in preheated oven about 20 minutes or until browned. Makes 12 muffins.

Banana-Marmalade Muffins

These muffins are moist and delicious. Serve with jam for breakfast. (Photo on page 44.)

1 cup all-purpose flour
2 teaspoons baking powder
1/2 teaspoon salt
1/2 teaspoon baking soda
1 teaspoon ground cinnamon
1 cup whole-wheat flour
2 tablespoons unprocessed wheat bran
2 tablespoons light-brown sugar
2 medium-size bananas, mashed
   (about 1 cup)

1/4 cup lime or orange marmalade,
   finely chopped
1 egg, beaten
1 cup plain low-fat yogurt
1/4 cup vegetable oil
1 teaspoon grated lime peel or orange
   peel

Per muffin:
160 calories
2.2 grams fiber

Preheat oven to 400F (205C). Grease 12 (2-1/2-to 3-inch) muffin cups. Sift all-purpose flour, baking powder, salt, baking soda and cinnamon into a medium-size bowl. Stir in whole-wheat flour, wheat bran and brown sugar; set aside. In another medium-size bowl, combine bananas, marmalade, egg, yogurt, oil and lime peel. Stir banana mixture into dry ingredients just until ingredients are moistened. Spoon batter into muffin cups, filling each 2/3 full. Bake in preheated oven about 20 minutes or until browned. Makes 12 muffins.

Cranberry-Bran Muffins

Your family will rave about these muffins. Serve for breakfast or as an after school snack.

2 cups All-Bran or Fiber One cereal
1-1/2 cups low-fat milk
1 cup cranberries, finely chopped
2 tablespoons sugar
2 cups all-purpose flour

1 tablespoon baking powder
1/4 teaspoon salt
1/4 cup honey
2 tablespoons vegetable oil
1 egg, beaten
1 teaspoon vanilla extract

Preheat oven to 400F (205C). Line 12 (2-1/2- to 3-inch) muffin cups with paper cups or spray with nonstick vegetable spray. In a medium-size bowl, combine cereal and milk. Let stand, stirring occasionally, 10 minutes or until cereal is softened. In a small bowl, combine cranberries and sugar; set aside. Sift flour, baking powder and salt into a medium-size bowl. Stir honey, oil, egg, vanilla and cranberry mixture into cereal mixture. Stir in dry ingredients just until moistened. Spoon batter into prepared muffin cups, filling each 2/3 full. Bake in preheated oven about 20 minutes or until muffins spring back when lightly pressed. Serve warm. Makes 12 muffins.

Per muffin:
152 calories
5.4 grams fiber

Variation
Date-Bran Muffins: Substitute 1/2 cup finely chopped dates for cranberries. Omit sugar.

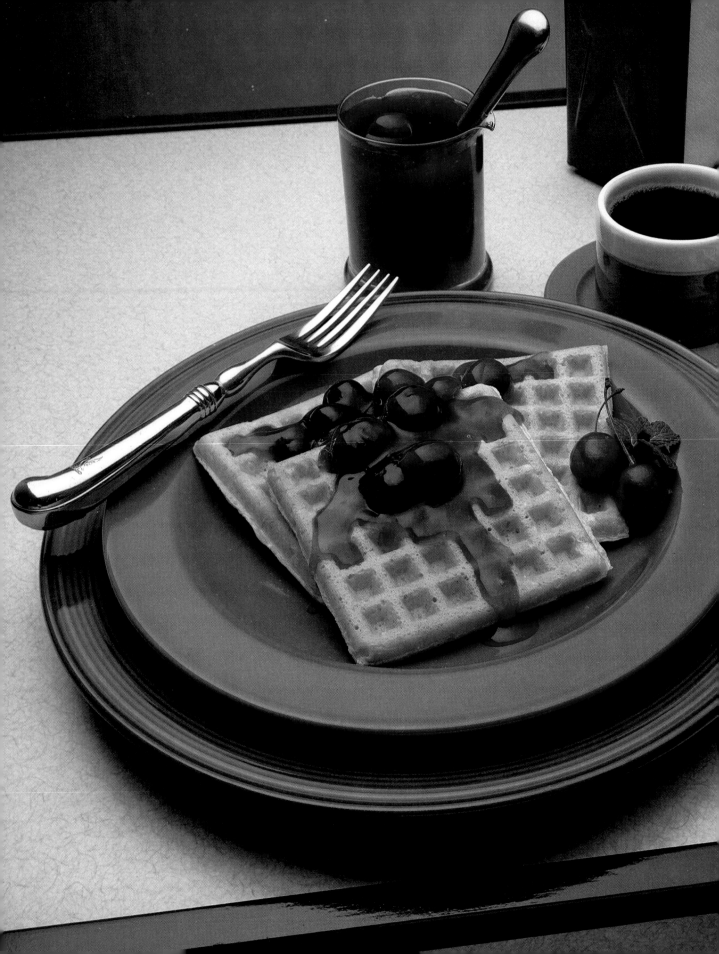

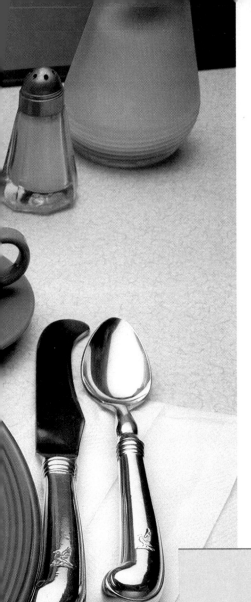

Cherry Sauce, page 130; Whole-Wheat Waffles, page 129

Breakfast & Brunch

CHAPTER EIGHT

Breakfast
& Brunch

Breakfast is one of the most neglected meals of the day; it is also one of the most important. It's a long time from dinner to lunch the next day; your body functions more efficiently if you provide it with a nourishing breakfast.

But you say that you don't like breakfast? You don't have to serve traditional breakfast fare each morning; choose a breakfast to suit you! A cup of hot soup or a peanut butter sandwich is okay. Some teenagers even eat leftover pizza—cold!

No time to cook? Prepare Whole-Wheat Waffles, page 129, and freeze them individually. Pop them into the toaster while you pour some juice. Make Fruitty-Nutty Yogurt, page 130, the night before for breakfast on the run.

One of my favorites is My Muesli, page 132. I keep it in a plastic container in the refrigerator. It's an easy breakfast for camping, too. Just take along some milk and fresh fruit for an easy and satisfying breakfast! You can even place each serving in a small plastic bag, add milk and eat—there're no dishes to wash.

Of course, everyone's favorite breakfasts are on weekends when there's more time for a leisurely meal—and more time to prepare it. Try No-Crust Quiche, page 135; it's easy because there's no crust to prepare. With fresh fruit, toasted Sesame-Oat Bread, page 112; and your favorite beverage, you have a complete meal.

These are only a few of the many possible suggestions. Try others in this chapter for new family favorites.

Blueberry-Oat Pancakes

Try these absolutely delicious pancakes! Serve with maple or blueberry syrup.

1-1/4 cups all-purpose flour
1-1/2 teaspoons baking powder
1/2 teaspoon baking soda
1/4 teaspoon salt
3/4 cup regular rolled oats
1 tablespoon light-brown sugar

1 tablespoon wheat germ
1 egg
2 cups plain low-fat yogurt
2 tablespoons vegetable oil
1 cup fresh or thawed frozen blueberries

Sift flour, baking powder, baking soda and salt into a medium-size bowl. Stir in oats, brown sugar and wheat germ; set aside. In a small bowl, lightly beat egg; stir in yogurt and oil. Preheat a nonstick griddle over medium heat. Stir liquid ingredients into dry ingredients until moistened. Gently stir in blueberries. Lightly grease griddle or spray with nonstick coating. Using about 1/3 cup for each pancake, pour pancake batter onto hot griddle. Cook until bubbles form in batter; turn. Cook until lightly browned on underside, about 2 minutes. Makes about 10 (5-inch) pancakes.

**Per pancake:
161 calories
1.8 grams fiber**

Whole-Wheat Waffles

Leftovers can be frozen and reheated in a toaster or oven. (Photo on page 126.)

1 cup all-purpose flour
2-1/2 teaspoons baking powder
1/2 teaspoon baking soda
1/4 teaspoon salt
3/4 cup whole-wheat flour

1/4 cup oat bran
2-1/2 cups buttermilk
1 egg, beaten
2 tablespoons vegetable oil

Preheat a waffle iron. Sift all-purpose flour, baking powder, baking soda and salt into a medium-size bowl. Stir in whole-wheat flour and oat bran; set aside. In a small bowl, combine buttermilk, egg and oil. Add buttermilk mixture to dry ingredients; stir until combined. Spoon into a waffle iron and bake according to manufacturer's directions until lightly browned. Makes 4 (8-inch-square) waffles.

**Per waffle:
179 calories
2.0 grams fiber**

Cherry Sauce

Delicious over waffles, pancakes or ice cream. Keep frozen cherries on hand to make this easy sauce. (Photo on page 126.)

1 tablespoon sugar or to taste
2 tablespoons cornstarch
1 cup unsweetened apple juice or water

1 cup frozen sweet dark cherries
1 teaspoon grated lemon peel

In a medium-size saucepan, combine sugar and cornstarch. Gradually stir in apple juice. Cook, stirring constantly, over medium heat until mixture is bubbly and slightly thickened. Stir in cherries and lemon peel; cook until heated through. Serve warm. Makes about 2 cups.

Blueberry-Orange Sauce

Try this on Whole-Wheat Waffles, page 129

1 tablespoon sugar or to taste
2 teaspoons cornstarch
1 cup orange juice or water

1-1/2 cups fresh or frozen blueberries
1 medium-size orange, peeled, sectioned
1 teaspoon grated orange peel

In a medium-size saucepan, combine sugar and cornstarch. Gradually stir in orange juice. Cook, stirring constantly, over medium heat until bubbly and slightly thickened. Stir in blueberries, orange and orange peel. Serve warm. Makes about 3 cups.

Variation
Maple, Blueberry & Orange Sauce: Add 1 cup maple syrup to warm sauce. Heat through. Makes about 4 cups.

Fruity-Nutty Yogurt

Serve for breakfast or as a snack.

1 quart plain low-fat yogurt
2 cups fresh or thawed frozen fruit in
   bite-sized pieces (strawberries,
   blueberries, raspberries, peaches,
   apricots, etc., or a combination)

1/4 cup chopped almonds or pecans
1/4 cup honey or to taste
1 teaspoon vanilla extract

Place yogurt in a medium-size bowl. Stir in fruit, nuts, honey and vanilla. Cover and refrigerate at least 2 hours or up to 12 hours. Stir before serving. Makes 6 servings.

Dates & Oat Bran

The dates add sweetness so more sugar is not needed. Recipe can be doubled or tripled. Serve with skim or low-fat milk.

1/3 cup oat bran
Dash salt

1 cup water
3 dates, pitted, finely chopped

In a small saucepan, combine oat bran, salt and water. Bring to a boil, stirring constantly. Stir in dates. Reduce heat to low. Cook, stirring constantly, 1 to 2 minutes or to desired thickness. Makes 1 serving.

**Per serving
191 calories
6.6 grams fiber**

Variation
Substitute 2 tablespoons chopped dried apricots or 3 tablespoons raisins for dates.

Creamy Rolled Oats

Because the milk is cooked with the oats, you don't add more milk—this keeps the cereal hot.

2/3 cup regular rolled oats
2/3 cup nonfat dry milk powder

Dash salt
2 cups water

In a medium-size saucepan, combine oats, dry milk powder, salt and water. Bring to a boil, stirring constantly, over medium heat. Boil 1 minute, stirring constantly. Remove from heat, cover and let stand about 2 minutes before serving. Makes 2 servings.

**Per serving
194 calories
2.7 grams fiber**

Variation
Stir in 1/2 cup chopped figs and 1/4 teaspoon cinnamon after mixture comes to a boil.

My Muesli

This is my version of a popular Swiss cereal. Vary the grains, fruits and nuts to come up with your favorite combination. Serve with fresh fruit and lots of milk or yogurt.

2 cups regular rolled oats
1 cup barley flakes
1 cup rye flakes
1 cup raisins
1/3 cup chopped dates or date morsels

3 cups wheat germ
2/3 cup diced dried fruit mix
1 (2-oz.) package almonds, finely
   chopped

Per serving:
205 calories
3.55 grams fiber

In a medium-size bowl, combine oats, barley and rye flakes, raisins, dates, wheat germ, dried fruit mix and nuts. Store in a plastic bag or a tightly covered container. Refrigerate up to 1 month or freeze up to 3 months. Makes 8 servings.

Apple Rings

Wonderful with toast and turkey sausage. These will be a breakfast favorite.

1 tablespoon butter or margarine
2 large Granny Smith apples, cored, cut
   crosswise in 1/4-inch rings

3 tablespoons honey or to taste
1/2 teaspoon ground allspice or
   cardamom

Per serving:
152 calories
1.9 grams fiber

In a large nonstick skillet, melt butter over medium heat. Add apples; turn to coat with butter. Reduce heat, cover and cook about 15 minutes or until apples are tender. Drizzle with honey; cook until apples are slightly caramelized. Sprinkle with allspice. Serve warm. Makes 2 to 3 servings.

Southwestern Breakfast Bake

Triple this hearty dish for a larger group. Serve with additional tortillas.

4 (6-inch) corn tortillas
1 (1-lb.) can vegetarian-style refried beans or "Refried" Beans, page 99

2 eggs
1 cup Salsa, page 31
1/4 cup (1 oz.) shredded Cheddar cheese

Preheat oven to 350F (175C). Lightly grease 2 (5-inch) round baking dishes. Wrap 2 tortillas in foil; set aside. Place 1 tortilla in bottom of each dish. Spoon 1/2 of beans on each tortilla. Using back of a spoon, make a slight hollow in center of beans. Break 1 egg into each hollow. Top each egg with 1/2 cup salsa. Sprinkle each dish with 1/2 of cheese. Bake about 20 minutes or until eggs are cooked to desired doneness. Place foil-wrapped tortillas in oven to warm during last 5 minutes of baking. Makes 2 servings.

> **Per serving:**
> **346 calories**
> **2.9 grams fiber**

Egg Bake

Baked eggs are a wonderful way to start the day!

1-1/4 pounds baking potatoes, peeled, coarsely chopped
1/2 cup low-fat milk
1/2 cup (2 oz.) shredded Cheddar cheese
Salt
White pepper

1/8 teaspoon freshly grated nutmeg or to taste
1 (10-oz.) package frozen chopped spinach, cooked, drained
4 eggs

In a medium saucepan, cook potatoes in boiling salted water about 20 minutes or until fork-tender. Drain; mash. Beat in milk and cheese. Season with salt, white pepper and nutmeg. Stir in spinach. Preheat oven to 400F (205C). Lightly grease a shallow 1-quart casserole dish. Spoon potato mixture into greased dish. Using back of a spoon, make 4 slight hollows in potato mixture. Break eggs into hollows. Bake in preheated oven about 20 minutes or until eggs are cooked to desired doneness. Makes 4 servings.

> **Per serving:**
> **180 calories**
> **2.2 grams fiber**

Spinach Frittata

This frittata combines whole eggs and egg whites to reduce the fat and cholesterol.

3 eggs
3 egg whites
1/2 cup (2 oz.) part-skim mozzarella
  cheese
1/4 teaspoon freshly grated nutmeg
Salt

Freshly ground pepper
1 (10-oz.) package frozen chopped
  spinach, thawed, well drained
1 tablespoon olive oil
1 small onion, chopped

Herbed Tomato Sauce:
1 (28-oz.) can crushed Italian tomatoes
1 cup beef stock
1 tablespoon red-wine vinegar
1 teaspoon dried leaf basil

1/2 teaspoon dried leaf oregano
Salt
Freshly ground pepper

Prepare sauce; keep warm or reheat when needed. In a medium-size bowl, lightly beat eggs, egg whites, cheese and nutmeg. Season with salt and pepper. Stir in spinach; set aside. In a 10-inch nonstick skillet, heat olive oil over medium heat. Add onion; sauté until softened. Using a slotted spoon, remove onion; stir into egg mixture. Pour egg mixture into skillet. Cook about 4 minutes or until bottom is lightly browned. Place a large plate over frittata. Invert frittata onto plate. Return frittata, uncooked side down, to skillet. Cook 3 to 4 minutes more or until cooked through. Cut in 6 wedges. Serve with sauce. Makes 6 servings.

Herbed Tomato Sauce:
In a medium-size saucepan, combine tomatoes, stock, vinegar, basil and oregano. Season with salt and pepper. Bring to a boil. Reduce heat, cover and simmer 30 minutes. If mixture is too thin, uncover and boil 5 minutes. Serve warm. Makes about 3 cups.

No-Crust Quiche

An easy, no-crust quiche that is tangy and delicious.

3 green onions, thinly sliced
1 small zucchini, shredded
1/2 cup (4 oz.) crumbled goat cheese
2 tablespoons grated Parmesan cheese
Freshly ground pepper
1/2 cup unbleached all-purpose flour

1/4 cup whole-wheat flour
3/4 teaspoon baking powder
1 tablespoon butter or margarine,
  chilled
1-1/2 cups low-fat milk
3 eggs

Preheat oven to 350F (175C). Lightly grease a 10-inch pie pan. Sprinkle onions and zucchini in greased pie pan. Top with cheeses. Season with pepper. In a blender or food processor fitted with the metal blade, combine flours and baking powder. Add butter; process 30 seconds or until butter is incorporated. Add milk and eggs; process 30 seconds or until blended. Pour over vegetables and cheeses. Bake about 30 minutes or until puffed and a knife inserted slightly off-center comes out clean. Serve hot. Makes 6 servings.

Per serving:
220 calories
1.4 grams fiber

Whole-Wheat Crepes

These crepes are slightly harder to cook than regular crepes because they are very tender and fragile.

2-1/4 cups low-fat milk
2 cups whole-wheat flour
3 eggs

2 tablespoons vegetable oil
1/8 teaspoon salt

In a blender, place milk, flour, eggs, oil and salt. Blend about 1 minute. Scrape down side of container; blend about 30 seconds. Let stand, covered, at room temperature 1 hour. Preheat a well-seasoned or nonstick 7-inch crepe pan over medium heat. Blend batter about 10 seconds; bran from whole-wheat flour will settle to bottom. Brush pan with oil or spray with nonstick coating. Pour 1/4 cup of batter into pan, tilting pan quickly so batter covers bottom completely. Cook until bottom of crepe is browned. Turn carefully as crepes are fragile. Brown other side a few seconds. Remove from pan. Repeat with remaining batter, adding oil or spraying as needed. Makes about 25 (6- to 7-inch) crepes.

Per crepe:
62 calories
0.9 gram fiber

Crab-Filled Crepes

Quick and delicious, these crepes make a perfect brunch treat. If the crepes are made ahead, the dish goes together in minutes.

1 tablespoon cornstarch
1 tablespoon all-purpose flour
1 cup chicken broth
1 cup low-fat milk
12 ounces crabmeat, flaked
1 (10-oz.) package frozen green peas,
  cooked

2 tablespoons chopped chives
1 tablespoon chopped fresh parsley
1 tablespoon lemon juice
8 Whole-Wheat Crepes, page 135
1/2 cup (2 oz.) shredded Swiss cheese

Spray a flameproof baking pan with nonstick cooking spray. Position oven rack about 6 inches from heat source; preheat broiler. To make filling, in a medium-size saucepan, combine cornstarch, flour and 1/4 cup of broth. Gradually stir in remaining broth and milk. Cook, stirring constantly, over medium heat until thickened and bubbly, about 5 minutes. Stir in crabmeat, peas, chives, parsley and lemon juice. Spoon about 1/2 cup of filling along 1 edge of each crepe; roll to enclose filling. Place crepes, seam-side down, in prepared pan. Sprinkle with cheese. Broil in preheated broiler until cheese melts, about 4 minutes. Makes 4 servings.

Variation
Chicken-Filled Crepes: Substitute 12 ounces chopped cooked chicken for crab and 1 pound cooked fresh asparagus, chopped, for peas.

Cranberry Coffeecake

Moist and flavorful, this coffeecake contains both soluble and insoluble fiber. (Photo on page 121.)

1 cup regular rolled oats
1 cup All-Bran with Extra Fiber or Fiber
    One cereal
1/4 cup butter or margarine
1/2 cup honey
2-1/4 cups boiling water
1 cup regular rolled oats
1/2 cup all-purpose flour
1/4 cup butter or margarine, chilled
1 cup dates, finely chopped

1 (12-oz.) package cranberries, coarsely
    chopped
1/2 cup sugar
2 cups all-purpose flour
1 tablespoon baking powder
1/2 teaspoon baking soda
1/4 teaspoon salt
1 teaspoon ground allspice
1 egg, beaten

In a medium-size bowl, combine 1 cup oats, cereal, 1/4 cup butter, honey and water. Let stand until cooled to room temperature, about 30 minutes, stirring occasionally. Preheat oven to 350F (175C). Spray a 13" x 9" baking pan with nonstick cooking spray. In another medium-size bowl, combine 1 cup oats and 1/2 cup flour. With a pastry blender or 2 knives, cut chilled butter into flour mixture until mixture resembles coarse crumbs. Stir in dates; set aside. In a small bowl, combine cranberries and sugar; set aside. Sift flour, baking powder, baking soda, salt and allspice into another medium-size bowl. Stir egg into cooled cereal mixture. Stir dry ingredients into cereal mixture just until combined. Spread 1/2 of batter in greased pan. Spoon 1/2 of cranberries over batter; sprinkle with 1/2 of date mixture. Repeat with remaining batter, cranberries and date mixture. Bake in preheated oven about 40 minutes or until cake springs back when lightly pressed. Cool slightly in pan on a wire rack. Cut into 18 bars. Serve warm or at room temperature. Makes 18 bars.

Per bar:
285 calories
4.0 grams fiber

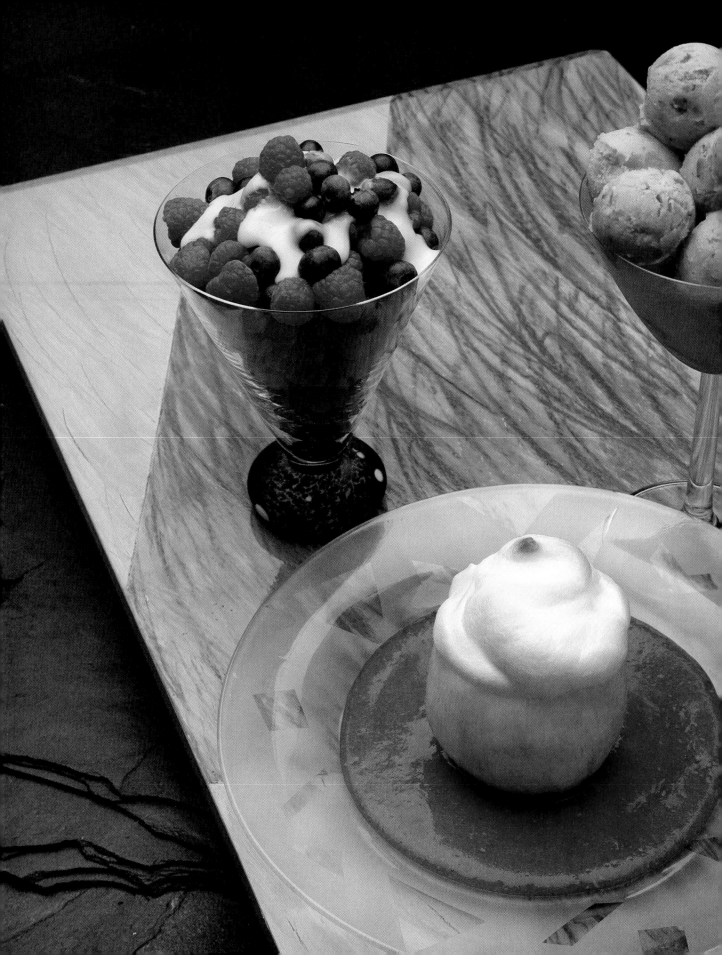

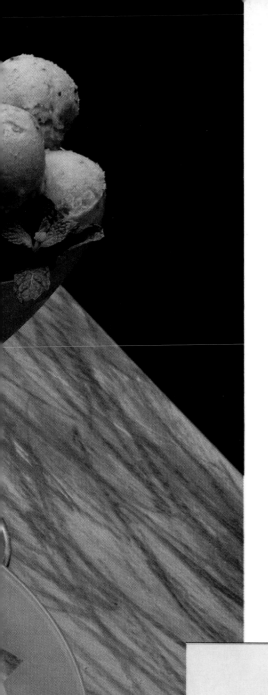

Clockwise from top left: Creamy Berry Dessert, page 144; Rhubarb-Strawberry Ice, page 150; Peach Alaska, page 142

Desserts

CHAPTER NINE

Desserts

Yes, even desserts can be delicious AND full of wholesome goodness! These desserts are lower in fat and sugar, which makes them lower in calories, too. Fruits are used extensively in dishes, such as Creamy Berry Dessert, page 144; Mango Sorbet, page 151; and Peach Alaska, page 142, but not all of the desserts contain fruit. Some desserts, such as Upside Down Rhubarb-Strawberry Jam Cake, page 148; and Sweet-Potato Custard, page 144, use fiber-rich vegetables for flavor. Chocolate lovers have not been neglected—even confirmed chocoholics will rave about Fudgy Oatmeal Brownies, page 155. The fiber in these desserts is from oats, whole-wheat flour and the fruits and vegetables.

Many of the desserts are modified versions of traditional ones that our grandmothers made—desserts with lots of fresh ingredients, love and comfort. These reflect a trend toward keeping regional foods alive, but sometimes changing them to fit today's lifestyle.

Desserts can be used as snacks or as the finishing touch to a meal. Some, such as Applesauce-Fig Bars, page 156; or Spicy Zucchini Cake, page 148, travel well and are great treats for a brown-bag lunch. When choosing desserts for a meal, consider the other courses that are to be served. Choose a light dessert, such as Rhubarb-Strawberry Ice, page 150, to follow a filling main dish. Blackberry Dumplings, page 154, would be the perfect ending to a light meal.

Enjoy!

Double Strawberry Tarts

Beautiful to look at, and just wait until you taste it!

2 cups fresh or frozen strawberries
2 tablespoons sugar
2 teaspoons cornstarch
6 baked Brown-Sugar & Almond
  Meringue Shells, below

3 cups Rhubarb-Strawberry Ice,
  page 150

In a food processor fitted with the metal blade, process strawberries to a puree; set aside. In a medium-size saucepan, combine sugar and cornstarch. Gradually stir in 1/4 cup of strawberry puree, then stir in remaining puree. Cook, stirring constantly, over medium heat until mixture is slightly thickened. Cool strawberry sauce to room temperature. Place a meringue shell on each of 6 dessert plates. Scoop Rhubarb-Strawberry Ice into shells. Drizzle sauce over ice. Makes 6 servings.

Per serving:
325 calories
2.7 grams fiber

Brown-Sugar & Almond Meringue Shells

Less delicate than the usual meringue shells, these have a nutty flavor that is very appealing. The brown sugar should be moist and free from lumps. If meringue edges start to brown, reduce oven temperature to 250F (120C).

4 egg whites, room temperature
1/2 cup powdered sugar, sifted
1/4 cup packed light-brown sugar
1/2 (2-oz.) package blanched almonds,
  finely ground

1/4 cup regular rolled oats
1 teaspoon vanilla extract

Preheat oven to 300F (150C). Line 2 baking sheets with waxed paper. Draw 6 (5-inch) circles on waxed paper. In a medium-size bowl, beat egg whites until soft peaks form. Gradually beat in powdered sugar and brown sugar; beat until stiff and glossy. Fold in almonds, oats and vanilla. Divide mixture among 6 circles. Using back of a spoon, make a slight hollow in center of each egg-white circle. Bake in preheated oven about 1-1/2 hours or until dry and crisp. Cool on a wire rack; remove from waxed paper. Store in an airtight container. Makes 6 meringue shells.

Per meringue:
115 calories
0.6 gram fiber

Peach Alaska

Pretty as a picture, this tastes as good as it looks! (Photo on page 139.)

2 large fresh peaches, peeled, halved,
    dipped in lemon juice
1/2 pint peach sorbet

4 egg whites, room temperature
1/2 cup powdered sugar

Raspberry Sauce:
2 cups fresh or thawed frozen
    raspberries
1 tablespoon sugar

1 tablespoon framboise (raspberry
    brandy), if desired

Prepare Raspberry Sauce; set aside. Preheat oven to 350F (175C). Fill each peach half with 1/4 of sorbet. Set in a baking pan; place in freezer while preparing meringue. In a medium-size bowl, beat egg whites until soft peaks form. Gradually beat in powdered sugar until egg whites are stiff and glossy. Remove peaches from freezer. Completely cover sorbet with meringue, sealing meringue to peaches. Place peaches on a baking sheet. Bake in preheated oven about 4 minutes or until meringue is golden brown. Spoon 1/4 of raspberry sauce into each of 4 dessert plates. Place a peach half on each plate in center of sauce. Serve immediately. Makes 4 servings.

Raspberry Sauce:
In a blender or food processor fitted with the metal blade, process raspberries, sugar and framboise, if desired, to a puree.

Mixed Fruit Crunch

This is a traditional dessert with new flavor combinations, or you can use your favorite fruits.

1 medium-size Granny Smith apple,
    cored, thinly sliced
4 nectarines, sliced
1 tablespoon lemon juice

1 cup fresh or thawed frozen blueberries
1/2 cup raisins
1/4 cup packed light-brown sugar

Topping:
1 cup regular rolled oats
1/4 cup all-purpose flour
1/4 cup packed light-brown sugar

1 tablespoon wheat germ
1/4 cup butter or margarine, melted
1 teaspoon vanilla extract

Preheat oven to 350F (175C). Grease an 8-inch-square baking pan. In a medium-size bowl, combine apple, nectarines and lemon juice. Stir in blueberries, raisins and brown sugar. Spoon into greased pan; set aside.

Prepare Topping; sprinkle over fruit mixture. Bake in preheated oven about 35 minutes or until apple is tender. Serve warm or at room temperature. Makes 6 servings.

Topping:
In a medium-size bowl, combine oats, flour, brown sugar and wheat germ. Stir in butter and vanilla until combined.

Oats & Berries

My version of a traditional Scottish dessert which is usually made with whipped cream.

1/2 cup regular rolled oats
2 cups plain low-fat yogurt
1/4 cup honey or to taste
1 teaspoon vanilla extract

1 cup chopped fresh or frozen
  strawberries
4 whole fresh strawberries, if desired

In a small heavy skillet, toast oats, stirring often, over medium heat until lightly browned. Cool to room temperature. In a medium-size bowl, combine yogurt, honey and vanilla. Stir in oats and chopped strawberries. Spoon into 4 serving dishes. Top each dessert with a whole strawberry, if desired. Serve immediately. Makes 4 servings.

**Per serving:
200 calories
2.0 grams fiber**

Variation
For a richer dessert, substitute 1/2 cup whipping cream, whipped, for 1 cup of yogurt.

Sweet-Potato Custard

Sweet-potato pie without the crust. Omitting the crust makes this dessert lower in calories.

1/3 cup granulated sugar
3 tablespoons water
1 (16-oz.) can sweet potatoes, drained
2 eggs
1/2 cup packed light-brown sugar

1-1/2 teaspoons ground cinnamon
1/2 teaspoon ground allspice
1/4 teaspoon ground cloves
1/4 teaspoon salt
1-1/2 cups low-fat milk

Preheat oven to 350F (175C). In a small saucepan, combine granulated sugar and water. Cook, stirring constantly, over medium-high heat until sugar caramelizes. Carefully pour hot syrup into a 1-quart soufflé dish. Quickly tilt dish to distribute syrup over bottom and part of side; set aside. In a food processor fitted with the metal blade, process sweet potatoes to a puree. Add eggs; process until combined. Add brown sugar, cinnamon, allspice, cloves and salt. Process until combined. With motor running, slowly add milk through feed tube. Place soufflé dish in a large deep pan. Pour custard mixture into dish. Pour enough boiling water around dish in pan to cover about half of dish. Bake in preheated oven about 50 minutes or until a knife inserted off-center comes out clean. Cool slightly. Cover and refrigerate until chilled. Makes 8 servings.

To make without food processor: In a large bowl, mash sweet potatoes. Beat in remaining ingredients in same order.

Creamy Berry Dessert

A summertime treat, this dessert is at its best with fresh berries. (Photo on page 139.)

1/3 cup sugar
1-1/2 tablespoons cornstarch
2 cups low-fat milk
2 eggs, beaten
1 teaspoon vanilla extract

2 tablespoons Grand Marnier or other orange-flavored liqueur
2 cups fresh or thawed frozen blueberries
1 cup fresh or thawed frozen raspberries

In a medium-size saucepan, combine sugar and cornstarch until blended. Gradually whisk in milk. Cook, stirring constantly, over medium heat until mixture comes to a boil. Boil 2 minutes, stirring constantly. Remove from heat. Beat 1/3 cup of mixture into eggs. Beat egg mixture into hot milk mixture. Cook, stirring constantly, about 2 minutes or until slightly thickened. Pour custard into a heatproof bowl; cool slightly. Stir in vanilla and

Grand Marnier. Cover surface with plastic wrap; refrigerate until chilled. Layer blueberries and raspberries in 4 glass serving dishes, reserving some of berries for garnish. Spoon chilled custard over berries. Garnish with reserved berries. Makes 4 servings.

Winter Fruit Compote

A make-ahead dessert, this is also delightful for a winter meal.

2 large navel oranges
1 (8-oz.) package dried mixed fruit
1-1/2 cups dry white wine

1/4 cup packed light-brown sugar
1 (3-inch) cinnamon stick
1/4 cup slivered almonds, if desired

Cut 1 (3-inch) orange-peel strip; grate 1 tablespoon orange peel. Set aside. Peel oranges, removing all bitter white pith. Section oranges. Place orange sections in a bowl, cover and refrigerate. In a medium-size saucepan, combine reserved orange-peel strip and grated peel, dried mixed fruit, wine, brown sugar and cinnamon stick. Bring to a boil. Reduce heat, cover and simmer about 15 minutes or until fruit is tender. Cool to room temperature. Pour into a serving bowl, cover and refrigerate until chilled. Discard cinnamon stick and orange peel. Stir in orange sections. Sprinkle with almonds, if desired. Makes 6 servings.

> **Per serving:**
> 180 calories
> 1.7 grams fiber

Apple Compote

Warm and comforting, compote is also delicious topped with creamy plain yogurt.

2 pounds Granny Smith apples, thinly
  sliced
1/2 cup orange marmalade

1/4 cup chopped dried apricots
1/2 cup dry white wine

Preheat oven to 350F (175C). Grease a 1-quart baking dish. Arrange apple slices in layers in greased dish. In a small bowl, combine marmalade, apricots and wine; pour over apples. Cover and bake in preheated oven about 35 minutes or until apples are tender. Serve warm or at room temperature. Makes 4 to 6 servings.

> **Per serving:**
> 277 calories
> 6.0 grams fiber

Variation
Substitute 1/4 cup honey for marmalade. Add 1/4 teaspoon ground cardamom.

Kentucky Apple Stack Cake

This traditional Kentucky cake is adapted from my aunt's recipe. She used home-dried apples, but commercially prepared ones work fine.

Cake:

2 cups all-purpose flour
1 tablespoon plus 1 teaspoon baking powder
1/2 teaspoon baking soda
2 cups whole-wheat flour
1/2 cup packed light-brown sugar

1/4 cup granulated sugar
1/2 cup butter or margarine, chilled
2 eggs, beaten
About 1 cup buttermilk
1/2 teaspoon vanilla extract
Powdered sugar

Spicy Apple Filling:

4 cups dried apples (1 lb.)
Water
1 cup packed dark-brown sugar

2-1/2 teaspoons ground cinnamon
3/4 teaspoon ground cloves
1/2 teaspoon ground allspice

Per serving:
269 calories
1.8 grams fiber

Cake: Preheat oven to 425F (220C). Turn 3 (9-inch) round cake pans upside down. Grease bottoms. Sift all-purpose flour, baking powder and baking soda into a medium-size bowl. Stir in whole-wheat flour and sugars. Using 2 knives or a pastry blender, cut in butter until mixture resembles coarse crumbs. Stir in eggs, buttermilk and vanilla to make a soft dough. Knead dough lightly on a floured board. Divide dough in 6 equal pieces. Pat each piece in a 9-inch circle. Place 1 circle on each greased pan bottom. Reserve remaining circles. Bake in preheated oven about 15 minutes or until centers spring back when lightly pressed. Remove from pans; cool on wire racks. Bake remaining dough circles; cool.

Filling:

In a large saucepan, combine apples and enough water to cover. Cook, stirring occasionally, over medium heat about 30 minutes or until apples are soft and water is absorbed. Add more water during cooking, if necessary. Stir apples frequently near end of cooking time to prevent burning. Mash apples. Stir in brown sugar and spices. Cool to room temperature.

To assemble:

Place 1 cake layer on a serving plate. Top with 1/5 of cooled filling. Repeat with remaining cake layers and filling, ending with a cake layer. Wrap and refrigerate overnight or up to 2 days before serving. To serve, sprinkle with powdered sugar. Makes 16 servings.

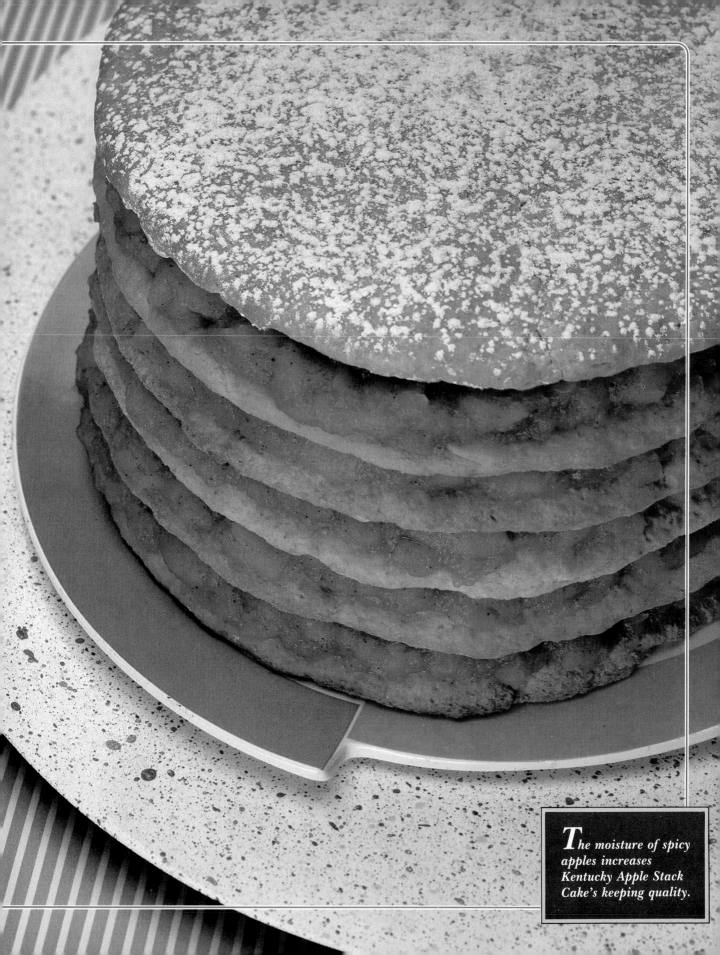

The moisture of spicy apples increases Kentucky Apple Stack Cake's keeping quality.

Spicy Zucchini Cake

Moist and delicious, this cake is excellent for packed lunches.

1 cup all-purpose flour
1-1/2 teaspoons baking powder
2 teaspoons baking soda
2 teaspoons ground cinnamon
1/4 teaspoon ground cloves
1/2 teaspoon salt
1 cup whole-wheat flour
3/4 cup granulated sugar

1/2 cup packed light-brown sugar
3/4 cup vegetable oil
2 eggs, beaten
1/2 cup low-fat milk
1 teaspoon vanilla extract
2 cups shredded zucchini
1 cup raisins

Per bar:
224 calories
1.8 grams fiber

Preheat oven to 350F (175C). Grease a 13" x 9" baking pan. Sift all-purpose flour, baking powder, baking soda, spices and salt into a medium-size bowl. Stir in whole-wheat flour and sugars, then oil, eggs, milk and vanilla. Beat with an electric mixer on medium speed 2 to 3 minutes or until blended. Stir in zucchini and raisins. Pour into greased pan. Bake in preheated oven 45 to 50 minutes or until a wooden pick inserted in center comes out clean. Cool in pan on a wire rack. Makes 18 (3" x 2") bars.

Upside Down Rhubarb-Strawberry Jam Cake

Rhubarb requires more sugar than is used for most recipes in this book. However, I think you'll agree that it's occasionally worth a few extra calories.

2 cups fresh or thawed frozen chopped
  rhubarb (8 oz.)
1/4 cup water
1/2 cup granulated sugar
1/2 cup all-purpose flour
1 teaspoon baking powder
1/2 teaspoon baking soda

1/2 cup whole-wheat flour
1/4 cup butter or margarine, room
  temperature
1/4 cup packed light-brown sugar
1 egg
1/3 cup strawberry jam
1/2 cup buttermilk

Per serving:
331 calories
1.6 grams fiber

Preheat oven to 350F (175C). Lightly grease a 9-inch-round cake pan. In a medium-size saucepan, combine rhubarb, water and granulated sugar. Bring to a boil. Reduce heat, cover and simmer until rhubarb is almost tender. Cool slightly. Pour into greased pan; set aside. Sift all-purpose flour, baking powder and baking soda into a medium-size bowl. Stir in whole-wheat flour; set aside. In a medium-size bowl, cream butter and brown sugar until light and fluffy. Add egg; beat 2 minutes. In a glass measuring cup, combine jam and buttermilk. Alternately stir dry ingredients and buttermilk mixture into brown sugar mixture. Pour over rhubarb. Bake in preheated oven about 45 minutes or until cake springs back when lightly pressed. Let cool in pan on a wire rack 10 minutes. Place a large plate over pan; invert. Let pan remain over cake about 5 minutes. Serve warm. Makes 8 servings.

Banana Cake

Look for oat bran in the cereal section of your supermarket. It adds a rich moistness and a subtle flavor as well as fiber.

1-1/2 cups all-purpose flour	2 eggs
1-1/2 teaspoons baking powder	2 medium-size very ripe bananas,
1/2 teaspoon baking soda	mashed (about 1 cup)
1/4 teaspoon salt	1/3 cup buttermilk
3/4 cup oat bran	1 teaspoon vanilla extract
1/2 cup vegetable oil	1/2 cup raisins
1 cup packed dark-brown sugar	1/2 cup chopped pecans

Creamy Frosting, if desired:

1 (8-oz.) package Neufchâtel cheese, room temperature	About 2 cups powdered sugar, sifted
	1 teaspoon vanilla extract

Preheat oven to 350F (175C). Grease a 13" x 9" baking pan. Sift flour, baking powder, baking soda and salt into a medium-size bowl. Stir in oat bran; set aside. In another medium-size bowl, combine oil, brown sugar, eggs, bananas, buttermilk and vanilla. Beat with an electric mixer until well mixed. Beat flour mixture into banana mixture until combined. Stir in raisins and nuts; pour into greased pan. Bake in preheated oven 25 to 30 minutes or until cake springs back when lightly pressed. Cool in pan on a wire rack. Frost with Creamy Frosting, if desired. Makes 18 (3" x 2") bars.

Per bar without frosting: 205 calories 1.1 grams fiber

Creamy Frosting:

In a small bowl, beat cheese until creamy. Beat in enough sugar for a good spreading consistency, then beat in vanilla.

Chocolate Pudding & Cake

Pudding on the bottom and moist cake on the top—what a delicious treat!

2/3 cup all-purpose flour
2 teaspoons baking powder
1/4 teaspoon salt
2 teaspoons unsweetened cocoa powder
1/2 cup packed light-brown sugar
1/3 cup oat bran
3/4 cup low-fat milk
2 tablespoons unsalted butter or
   margarine, room temperature

2 teaspoons vanilla extract
1/2 cup chopped walnuts
2/3 cup packed light-brown sugar
3 tablespoons unsweetened cocoa
   powder
1 cup boiling water

Preheat oven to 325F (165C). Sift flour, baking powder, salt and 2 teaspoons cocoa powder into a medium-size bowl. Stir in 1/2 cup brown sugar and oat bran. Add milk, butter and vanilla; beat until smooth, about 2 minutes. Stir in nuts. Pour batter into a 9-inch-square pan. In a small bowl, combine 2/3 cup brown sugar and 3 tablespoons cocoa powder. Sprinkle over batter. Carefully pour water over sugar mixture. Bake in preheated oven about 35 minutes or until top is firm to the touch. Serve warm. Makes 6 servings.

Rhubarb-Strawberry Ice

This has the flavors of springtime. Serve after a substantial meal as a light and refreshing finish. (Photo on page 139.)

2 cups fresh or thawed frozen chopped
   rhubarb (8 oz.)
1/4 cup water
1/2 cup sugar
2 cups fresh or frozen strawberries,
   coarsely chopped

2 tablespoons orange-flavored liqueur
2 cups low-fat milk
Fresh mint, if desired

In a small saucepan, cook rhubarb in water over medium heat about 10 minutes or until tender. Stir in sugar until dissolved. Cool to room temperature. In a medium-size bowl, combine strawberries and liqueur. Let stand 10 minutes. Stir in rhubarb mixture and milk. Freeze in an ice cream freezer according to manufacturer's directions. Or pour into a 9-inch-square pan. Freeze until almost solid, 1 to 3 hours. Scrap into a bowl. Beat with an electric mixer until fluffy. Pour back into pan; freeze until solid. To serve, garnish with mint, if desired. Makes about 4 cups.

Melon with Melon-Mint Sorbet

Refreshing as a light dessert or as a palate cleanser between courses. (Photo on page 153.)

1/2 cup packed mint leaves, chopped
1/2 cup water
2 tablespoons sugar
1/2 small cantaloupe, cubed

2 tablespoons melon-flavored liqueur, if desired
1 honeydew melon, cut in balls, chilled
Fresh mint, if desired

In a small saucepan, combine mint and water. Bring to a boil. Let stand 10 minutes. Using a fine strainer, strain liquid into a small bowl; discard mint leaves. Stir sugar into mint liquid until dissolved. Cover and refrigerate until chilled. In a food processor fitted with the metal blade, process cantaloupe to a puree. You should have about 2 cups puree. In a medium-size bowl, combine cantaloupe puree, mint liquid and liqueur, if desired. Freeze in an ice cream freezer according to manufacturer's directions. Or pour into a 9-inch-square pan. Freeze until almost solid, 1 to 3 hours. Scrape into a bowl; beat with an electric mixer until fluffy. Pour back into pan. Freeze until solid. To serve, spoon honeydew melon balls into 6 dessert dishes. Top with scoops of sorbet. Garnish with mint, if desired. Makes 6 servings.

Per serving:
98 calories
2.6 grams fiber

Variation
Melon-Orange Sorbet: Omit mint leaves and melon-flavored liqueur. Reduce water to 1/3 cup. In a small saucepan, bring sugar and water to a boil. Cover and refrigerate until chilled. Stir in 2 tablespoons orange-flavored liqueur. Continue as directed above.

Mango Sorbet

Cool and refreshing, this colorful sorbet has a taste of the tropics.

1/3 cup water
3 tablespoons sugar

2 (12-oz.) ripe mangos

In a small saucepan, combine water and sugar. Bring to a boil over medium heat, stirring to dissolve sugar. Cool to room temperature. Peel mangos. Cut pulp from seed; coarsely chop pulp. In a blender or food processor fitted with the metal blade, process mangos to a puree. Add cooled sugar syrup; process until combined. Freeze in an ice cream freezer according to manufacturer's directions. Or pour into a 9-inch-square pan. Freeze until almost solid, about 2 hours. Scrape into a bowl; beat with an electric mixer until fluffy. Pour back into pan; freeze until almost solid. Makes 4 servings.

Per serving:
75 calories
1.4 grams fiber

Fruit Fool

Low-fat yogurt and beaten egg whites substitute for the usual whipped cream.

2/3 cup pitted prunes (about 4 oz.)
4 canned pear halves, drained, cut in chunks
1/2 cup lemon-flavored low-fat yogurt

1 teaspoon grated lemon peel
1 egg white
Lemon-peel twists

Cook prunes according to package directions until tender. Drain; cool to room temperature. In a food processor fitted with the metal blade, process prunes and pears to a puree. Pour into a medium-size bowl. Stir in yogurt and grated lemon peel. In a small bowl, beat egg white until stiff but not dry. Fold into fruit mixture. Spoon into 4 dessert dishes. Decorate with lemon-peel twists. Makes 4 servings.

Variation
Substitute any well-drained cooked fruit for prunes and pears. Vary yogurt flavor to match fruit. Sweeten to taste with honey or sugar.

Blackberry Cobbler

This is one of my husband's favorite desserts.

2/3 cup sugar
2 tablespoons all-purpose flour

Crust:
1/2 cup all-purpose flour
1 teaspoon baking powder
1/2 cup whole-wheat flour

4 cups fresh or thawed frozen blackberries (1 lb.)

1-1/2 tablespoons butter or margarine, chilled
6 tablespoons low-fat milk

Preheat oven to 425F (220C). In a medium-size bowl, combine sugar and flour. Add berries; toss to combine. Pour into a 9-inch-square baking dish; set aside. Prepare Crust. Place dough over berries. Trim to fit, if necessary. Using point of a sharp knife, cut 3 (1-inch) slits in dough for steam to escape. Bake in preheated oven about 30 minutes or until crust is browned and filling is bubbly. Makes 6 servings.

Crust:
Sift all-purpose flour and baking powder into a small bowl. Stir in whole-wheat flour. Using 2 knives or a pastry blender, cut in butter until mixture resembles coarse crumbs. Stir in milk to make a soft dough. Turn out dough onto a lightly floured board. Knead lightly until smooth. Roll out dough to a 10-inch square.

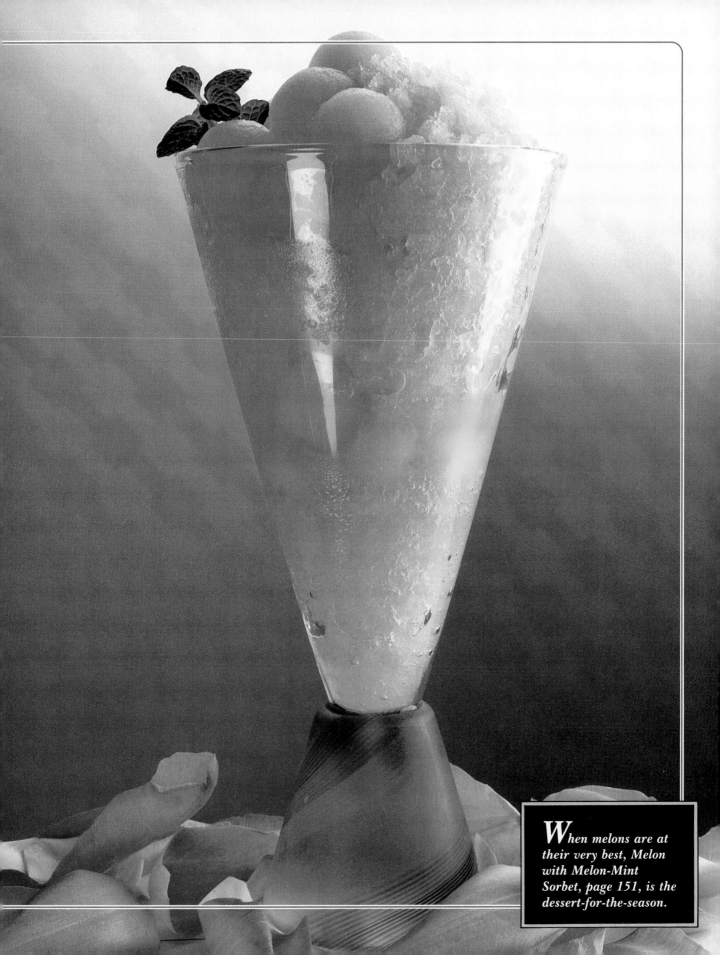

When melons are at their very best, Melon with Melon-Mint Sorbet, page 151, is the dessert-for-the-season.

Blackberry Dumplings

Dumplings are very traditional in the South. They can be made with almost any fruit.

1 cup all-purpose flour
1 tablespoon sugar
2-1/2 teaspoons baking powder
1/4 teaspoon salt
1 cup whole-wheat flour
3 tablespoons butter or margarine, chilled

3/4 cup low-fat milk
2-1/4 cups fresh or thawed frozen blackberries
1/2 cup plus 1 tablespoon sugar

Topping:
1/2 cup sugar
1 tablespoon all-purpose flour

1 cup water
1 tablespoon lemon juice

Per serving:
165 calories
2.7 grams fiber

Grease a 9-inch-square baking dish. Preheat oven to 400F (205C). Sift all-purpose flour, 1 tablespoon of sugar, baking powder and salt into a medium-size bowl. Stir in whole-wheat flour. Using 2 knives or a pastry blender, cut in butter until mixture resembles coarse crumbs. Stir in milk to make a soft dough. Turn out dough onto a lightly floured board. Knead lightly until smooth. Roll out dough to a 12-inch square. Cut in 9 (4-inch) squares. Spoon 1/4 cup blackberries into center of 1 square. Sprinkle with 1 tablespoon of sugar. Bring opposite corners of dough to center; seal edges. Place in greased dish. Repeat with remaining squares, berries and sugar. Prepare Topping; pour over dumplings. Bake in preheated oven about 30 minutes or until dumplings are lightly browned and crust is cooked through. Makes 9 servings.

Topping:

In a medium-size saucepan, combine sugar and flour. Gradually stir in water. Bring to a boil; boil 2 minutes. Remove from heat; stir in lemon juice.

Cherry Bread Pudding

This pudding is sure to make a hit. Fresh cherries can be used when they're in season.

2 cups thawed frozen dark sweet
   cherries, drained
3 whole-wheat bread slices, cut in 1-inch
   cubes
2 eggs
1/3 cup packed light-brown sugar

2 cups low-fat milk
1/4 cup sliced almonds
1 teaspoon vanilla extract
1/2 teaspoon ground cinnamon
1/4 teaspoon freshly grated nutmeg

Lightly grease a 9-inch-square baking dish. Combine cherries and bread in greased dish; set aside. In a medium-size bowl, beat eggs and sugar until light and foamy. Gradually beat in milk. Stir in almonds, vanilla, cinnamon and nutmeg. Pour over cherry mixture. Let stand about 30 minutes to soften bread. Preheat oven to 350F (175C). Bake in preheated oven about 50 minutes or until a knife inserted off-center comes out clean. Serve warm or at room temperature. Makes 6 servings.

**Per serving:
208 calories
1.0 gram fiber**

Variation
Substitute other well-drained fruit, such as peaches, plums or apricots, for cherries.

Fudgy Oatmeal Brownies

Wonderfully moist and fudgy, chocoholics will love these cake-like brownies.

1-1/2 cups boiling water
1 cup regular rolled oats
1 cup all-purpose flour
1/3 cup unsweetened cocoa powder
1 teaspoon baking soda
1/4 teaspoon salt

1/2 cup butter or margarine, melted
1/2 cup packed light-brown sugar
3/4 cup granulated sugar
2 eggs
1 teaspoon vanilla extract

Preheat oven to 350F (175C). Lightly grease a 13" x 9" baking pan. In a medium-size bowl, combine water and oats. Let stand until almost room temperature. Sift flour, cocoa powder, baking soda and salt into a medium-size bowl; set aside. In another medium-size bowl, beat butter, sugars, eggs and vanilla with an electric mixer until blended, about 2 minutes. Beat in cooled oats until combined. Add dry ingredients; beat until combined. Pour batter into greased pan. Bake in preheated oven about 25 minutes or until top springs back when lightly pressed. Cool in pan on a wire rack. Makes 16 (3-1/4" x 2-1/4") brownies.

**Per brownie:
145 calories
0.9 gram fiber**

Applesauce-Fig Bars

Triticale is a grain developed by crossing wheat and rye. It has some characteristics of each. Its amino acid balance is better than either wheat or rye, but it is low in gluten.

1 cup all-purpose flour
1-1/4 teaspoons baking powder
3/4 teaspoon baking soda
1 teaspoon ground cinnamon
1/4 teaspoon ground cloves
1/4 teaspoon salt
1 cup whole-wheat or triticale flour

1/2 cup butter or margarine, room
   temperature
2/3 cup packed light-brown sugar
1 egg
1 cup unsweetened applesauce
3/4 cup chopped dried figs
1/2 cup chopped pecans

Preheat oven to 350F (175C). Grease a 13" x 9" baking pan. Sift all-purpose flour, baking powder, baking soda, cinnamon, cloves and salt into a medium-size bowl. Stir in whole-wheat flour; set aside. In another medium-size bowl, beat butter and brown sugar until light and fluffy, then beat in egg. Stir in applesauce. Beat in flour mixture; beat 2 minutes. Stir in figs and nuts. Pour into greased pan. Bake in preheated oven about 25 minutes or until top springs back when lightly pressed. Makes 24 (3" x 1-1/2") bars.

Variation

Spread with **Applesauce Frosting:** In a small bowl, beat 1 cup powdered sugar, 2 ounces Neufchâtel cheese and 2 teaspoons unsweetened applesauce until creamy.

Metric Chart

Comparison to Metric Measure

When You Know	Symbol	Multiply By	To Find	Symbol
teaspoons	tsp	5.0	milliliters	ml
tablespoons	tbsp	15.0	milliliters	ml
fluid ounces	fl. oz.	30.0	milliliters	ml
cups	c	0.24	liters	l
pints	pt.	0.47	liters	l

When You Know	Symbol	Multiply By	To Find	Symbol
quarts	qt.	0.95	liters	l
ounces	oz.	28.0	grams	g
pounds	lb.	0.45	kilograms	kg
Fahrenheit	F	5/9 (after subtracting 32)	Celsius	C

Liquid Measure to Liters

1/4 cup	=	0.06 liters
1/2 cup	=	0.12 liters
3/4 cup	=	0.18 liters
1 cup	=	0.24 liters
1-1/4 cups	=	0.3 liters
1-1/2 cups	=	0.36 liters
2 cups	=	0.48 liters
2-1/2 cups	=	0.6 liters
3 cups	=	0.72 liters
3-1/2 cups	=	0.84 liters
4 cups	=	0.96 liters
4-1/2 cups	=	1.08 liters
5 cups	=	1.2 liters
5-1/2 cups	=	1.32 liters

Fahrenheit to Celsius

F	C
200—205	95
220—225	105
245—250	120
275	135
300—305	150
325—330	165
345—350	175
370—375	190
400—405	205
425—430	220
445—450	230
470—475	245
500	260

Liquid Measure to Milliliters

1/4 teaspoon	=	1.25 milliliters
1/2 teaspoon	=	2.5 milliliters
3/4 teaspoon	=	3.75 milliliters
1 teaspoon	=	5.0 milliliters
1-1/4 teaspoons	=	6.25 milliliters
1-1/2 teaspoons	=	7.5 milliliters
1-3/4 teaspoons	=	8.75 milliliters
2 teaspoons	=	10.0 milliliters
1 tablespoon	=	15.0 milliliters
2 tablespoons	=	30.0 milliliters

INDEX